Here's what readers are saying about The Body Sculpting Bible for Men

I'm in week three of your advanced program. What a great program! At 46 years old, I've led a healthy lifestyle for many years and have been working out for 25-plus years...The first two weeks on your programs, I've seen distinct changes in my body. More muscle definition and greater muscle size.

—David D.

I just wanted to send a big thank you for your fantastic book. I have been on this program for just a few weeks now, and I've already seen big differences! Thank you so much for putting out such a COMPLETE and thorough book. I do not know of any other one source that puts together so much great and necessary detail.

Keep up the great work. You've already made a big difference in my life. I also recently bought the Power Block dumbbells on your recommendation and I love them, too!

—Rob V. (Lake Forest, Calif.)

I started your program six weeks ago, and I am in the best shape of my life. I used the 14-day Body Sculpting Workout #2 and it has given me incredible results! You guys have done a great job of informing and motivating the reader for a great routine. Again, this book was a revelation to me in many ways. I feel like this book cuts straight to the point in a fresh, straightforward way.

—Michael F.

This is one of the most informative fitness books I have ever laid my eyes on. I have used this book to change my entire work out. The photographs are amazing. Detail, Detail, Detail. This Is A Must BUY...

—Richard B.

I have been following this book for 2 months and I have never felt better. I have learned a lot and turned my wife on to the woman edition and she follows it and loves it. Thanks!

—A reader from Ft. Myers, Fla.

This book addressed exactly what I was looking for. All the exercises are thoroughly detailed and they explain the mistakes that you should avoid while performing them. The majority of the exercises described in the book are done with free weights, so machines are not required. Almost all of the workouts can be done at home with a basic dumbbell set. I found the book's coverage of nutrition and fat burning extremely helpful. Workout charts and sample diets are also included, so you know exactly how to start. The book also covers all levels of body sculpting. I have already begun to see my body take shape and am very satisfied with this book.

—*A reader from Connecticut*

Great book! Easy to ready, covers the entire subject...workouts, nutrition, supplements, etc. I've been doing it for six weeks and have seen great results. The concept of the 14-day workout makes sense and allows for a schedule that can last a lifetime. I highly recommend this book!

—*A reader from Bordentown, N.J.*

I've been a personal trainer in New York City for the last eight years and have read countless books on the subject of fitness.

For the last two months I have implemented The Body Sculpting Bible techniques into my personal training programs and have seen truly impressive results with all of my clients.

No other book has provided me with such effective and useful tools that have helped me help my clients achieve great progress in such a short amount of time.

Because of this book, my personal training business has absolutely increased. If you're looking for a straightforward, realistic, and effective fitness book for men, this is a must read!

—*A reader from New York City*

These guys did an excellent job. The book is easy to understand, and rich in information and routines that anyone can follow. I've already read many books, but none of them is compared to The Body Sculpting Bible....If you were looking for a great fitness book, you've found it. Most importantly this 14 days program WORKS!

—*Norberto F. (Sao Paulo, Brazil)*

I wanted to start a weight-training program to finally get the body I wanted. I tend to try and research what I need to do before starting anything and this book was amazing. The mind to body connection helps with focusing on what muscles need to be exercised and keeping proper form in the movements. The nutrition information is excellent for the beginner with all the supplements out there it gives a wonderful easy to understand guide to what you should take to help get the body your looking for. The programs are easy to follow and detailed. The thing I like most about the book though is that it doesn't offer a quick fix—it gives you the foundation to start building a strong muscular body. So if you looking to start a new work out routine and to pack on muscle and take off the fat, I would highly recommend this book.

—*Lenny (Glendale, Ariz.)*

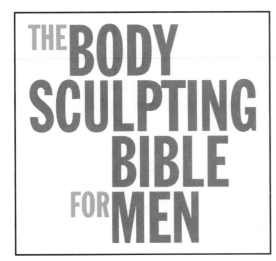

THE **BODY SCULPTING BIBLE** FOR **MEN**

Featuring the 14-Day Body Sculpting Workout

The Ultimate Fat Loss/Muscle Gain Program for the Ultimate Physique

**Written by:
James Villepigue
& Hugo A. Rivera**

**Photography by
Peter Field Peck**

Hatherleigh Press • New York

The Body Sculpting Bible For Men
A Hatherleigh Press/Getfitnow.com Book

Hatherleigh Press/Getfitnow.com Books
An Affiliate of W.W. Norton and Company, Inc.
5-22 46th Avenue, Suite 200
Long Island City, NY 11101
Toll Free 1-800-528-2550
Visit our websites getfitnow.com and hatherleighpress.com

Library of Congress Cataloging-in-Publication Data

Villepigue, James C.
   The body sculpting bible for men : featuring the 14-day body sculpting workout : the ultimate fat loss/muscle gain program for the ultimate physique / written by James Villepigue & Hugo A. Rivera ; photography by Peter Field Peck.
      p. cm.
   ISBN 1-57826-085-X (pbk. : alk. paper)
   1. Bodybuilding. I. Rivera, Hugo A., 1974-II. Title.

GV546.5 .V54 2001
646.7'5'081--dc21   2002019790

Disclaimer:
Before beginning any exercise program, consult your physician. The author and the publisher disclaim any liability, personal or professional, resulting from the application or misapplication of any of the information in this publication.

THE BODY SCULPTING BIBLE FOR MEN books are available for bulk purchase, special promotions and premiums. For more information on reselling and special purchase opportunities, please call us at 1-800-528-2550 and ask for the Special Sales Manager.

Cover Design by Angel Harleycat
Interior Design by Fatema Tarzi

10 9 8 7 6 5 4 3 2 1
Printed in Canada.

Dedications

This book is dedicated to my beautiful wife Lina who always loves and supports me unconditionally throughout any project, to my son Chad who is my pride and joy, to my parents and grandparents for always believing in me and who always ensured that I would get the best education possible as I was growing up, to my brother Raul whose computer knowledge made it possible for me to go online, to my in-laws who are always there to help me and provide me with support in time of need, and finally to God for giving me the talent to put this work together.

Hugo A. Rivera

Thank you God for giving me the strength, the courage and the confidence to overcome many of the dilemmas that we as humans must face in our lives. Thank you for helping me to achieve success and for keeping my faith strong, especially when I needed it most. I would like to dedicate these books first and foremost to my amazing parents Jim and Nancy, who happen to be the kindest, most loving and caring people I have ever had the pleasure of knowing. I love you both and appreciate every bit of love and guidance you have given me. To my extremely talented sister Deborah, who I am proud of and who I love more than she knows. To my wonderful grandparents Charles and Gloria, who are the most generous and selfless two people I know. I love you both!

To my beautiful girlfriend Stephanie, who happens to be the most dedicated and highly driven person I know. Thanks for pushing me when I didn't want to budge (I'm a Taurus you know!). I love you baby. And last but certainly not least, to all of our friends, clients and readers, thank you so much, for without you, we would not have had this great opportunity to share and pass along this refreshing and eye-opening knowledge of health and fitness.

James Villepigue

Special Thanks

Special thanks go out to:

Dr. Jack Barnathan, whose teachings were invaluable to the fine-tuning of this book.

Clark Bartram, for all of your priceless support, motivation and sincere kindness since the very beginning of this project.

Kurt Diekemper for giving me the necessary time off from work to enhance the quality of this work.

Dave Draper, for always leading by example and for being an inspiration to all who follow the body sculpting lifestyle.

Laree Draper for always being there to offer a hand.

Hatherleigh Press. Thank you so much, Andrew and Kevin, for giving us this great opportunity to share our knowledge and creativity with the world.

Robert Kennedy, for your commitment, faith and integrity during this project, and for being one of the nicest people and fitness leaders we've ever met.

The models, because words alone just wouldn't cut it: Arin Babaian, Ken Burke, Colin Burne, Dewayne Williams, James Carr.

Mike O'Hearn, for your time and generous contributions to this project.

Paragon Resorts, for allowing us to utilize your beautiful facilities for our photo shoots.

Peter Peck. Thank you so very much Peter! Your dedication, creativity and superb talent are invaluable and are greatly appreciated, brother.

Vickie Regnart, for graciously donating so much of her time to editing these pages, ensuring that this work would be what it is today.

Susan Ruszala, a true professional with great integrity and an extremely bright future. Thank you, Susan!

Rick Schaff. Thank you for your help, Rick! You have truly helped us avoid some major obstacles.

Fatema Tarzi, for all of the hard work, patience and sincerity that you've invested in this project. It is greatly appreciated!

Foreword

If you decided you wanted to build a house the first thing you would do after acquiring the land would be to hire an architect to make the blueprints for your future dream home. I also imagine that you would do your homework to find someone you really trust to design the biggest purchase of your lifetime. That process can be quite confusing and a bit frustrating because of the different styles and many options available in a market where there are so many qualified parties.

Once you have made your decision, you are "off to the races" as they say. The first thing you will receive from your architect (next to a whopping bill!) will be your own set of blueprints for your dream home. From there on in it is simply a matter of following those blueprints exactly, step by step, until the process is done. As hard as it is along the way, the end result will hopefully be one of joy and excitement as you enter your new home for the first time.

Let's imagine for a moment that you begin to doubt the process half way through the building process. You panic and get additional blueprints from the architect that was second on your list or your spouse says, "I told you this guy was better." The last thing you would do would be to abandon the original plan and start with the new ones. You would have a complete mess. Everything would fall apart and you would have wasted precious time and money along the way.

That is a simple analogy of what most people do when attempting to get in the best shape of their lives. I have competed for years and helped many others do the same. I have learned over the years that there are many good ways to get in shape. I would run if I heard someone touting that their system is "the best" or "the only way." We know in this industry that many people claim to be experts in the attempt to collect on innocent people looking for the so coveted "magic bullet." Guess what my friends? There is no such thing as a "magic bullet."

I am going to give you the bottom line; it takes work to get in shape. It also takes a plan. James Villepigue and Hugo Rivera have worked hard to lay out a time-tested plan of proper exercise, nutrition and supplementation coupled with consistency. They don't claim they have any new revelation or secret snake oil. They have done some homework and presented quality, time honored, information in an easy to understand format.

Another thing I have learned along the way is that people want results today. They become impatient so they abandon their original blueprint. If results don't come when they want, they automatically move to the next set of plans. When you combine systems and pick and choose what you like you dilute the plans all together. The one thing I advocate is to find a program you trust and stick it out until the end. The program laid out in this book will work. It will work if you apply the principles taught and follow through until the end. Don't abandon the plan halfway through. Don't let friends, experts, critics or anyone confuse your desire to attain better health through fitness.

Anyone involved in the fitness industry wants to help people; as health professionals we should collaborate in that single purpose. I might have a book someday and I would expect that others would advocate the use of the principles I choose to teach. By agreeing to write this foreword, I am acknowledging that I see James and Hugo desiring to help people get healthier and I am all for it.

Read the book; decide if the information is right for you and your goals. If it is, then by all means go for it! Take action today, make some positive changes and share the book with everyone you care about.

Clark Bartram
Host of American Health & Fitness

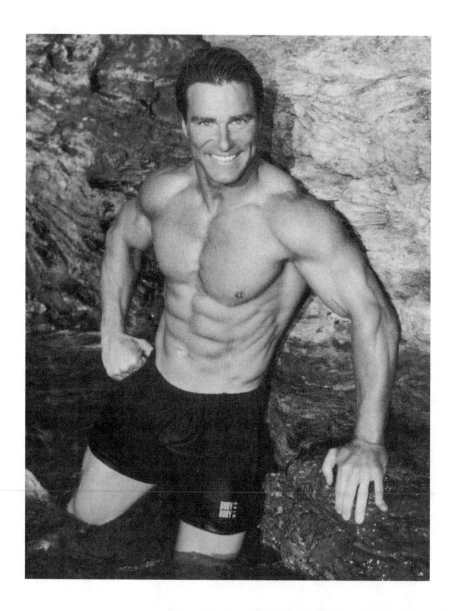

Preface

Everyone who has ever dedicated themselves to fitness or bodybuilding knows that there is no such thing as a "quick fix." Yet too often today the fitness programs available promise quick results with little work. The most effective bodybuilding techniques involve consistency in training and diet, good technique and form, and a commitment to getting in shape. The passion has to be there.

I have been passionately involved as a major influence in the fitness industry for many years now, as a publisher of *MuscleMag International* and in my youth as a participant in weightlifting and bodybuilding contests. *The Body Sculpting Bible* brings validity and a new sense of freshness to the fitness community by combining proven principles of training with a functional program that is geared to optimal results in today's hectic lifestyle.

The authors' 14-Day Body Sculpting Workout is a fantastic way for those who strive to reach peak physical condition and attain the body they desire. Yet *The Body Sculpting Bible* also offers easy-to-follow fitness programs for those who are just starting out. All of these programs combine weight lifting, aerobic exercise, sound nutrition and supplement programs, and strong motivational messages.

As an experienced fitness professional, I highly recommend this book to anyone who is interested in changing his or her physical appearance and fitness level from any starting point.

Robert Kennedy
Publisher, MuscleMag International

Quick Start

To get started with the *14-Day Body Sculpting Workout* as quickly as possible, follow the reading outline below. It will take you approximately 60 minutes at the most to go through this outline. We feel you'll need this basic understanding of the *14-Day Body Sculpting Workout* principles in order to harness the maximum benefits of the program.

Depending on your knowledge of how to perform the exercises, read the exercise descriptions that pertain to the routine that you choose.

We do recommend that you read through the entire book progressively to obtain the full benefits that the program has to offer. There is more than just training information in this book. This book will not only teach you how to change your physique, it will also teach you how to change your life!

Table of Contents

Precautions

Introduction

THE **BODY**
SCULPTING
BIBLE
FOR**MEN**

Every time we turn on the TV or read the latest muscle magazine we are bombarded with the latest way to lose fat, gain muscle and achieve the body of our dreams in only five minutes a day. We are constantly exposed to empty promises telling us that all we have to do to build a buff body is buy some fancy new machine (that may be as cheap as three small credit card installments of $75.99), take some new hyped up "magic" pill or go on a "new" diet, and that dream body will miraculously appear.

If you've ever bought one of those "body in a box" gadgets or machines, recall the process that took place when you received it. You used it for a few weeks, if at all, right? Eventually it ends up becoming a great place to lay your clothes. The only thing that ends up losing weight in this case is our wallet.

With so many diets, gadgets and magic potions available to us, it is no wonder that we become confused about how to properly get in shape. This is one of the major reasons why we decided to write this book. We are sick and tired of seeing and hearing about how people are ripped off by these "get fit quick" schemes and hokey solutions that provide nothing more than a healthy pile of junk. In addition, having dealt with weight problems throughout our youth, we naturally relate to people who want desperately to change the way they look and don't know how to go about doing so. We will show you that you can lose fat very easily without starving yourself. In fact, you may end up eating much more than you ever have in your life and still achieve the perfectly shaped physique you've been hoping for! We will also show you how to create lean muscle without having to exercise for hours a day. You don't even need to join a health club if you don't want to. Our goal is to share with you all of the knowledge that we have accumulated in our combined 20 years of bodybuilding experience. With this newfound knowledge you will soon be in total control of how you look and feel. No longer will it be a dreadful experience to step on the scale, try on those old jeans, put on that favorite suit that stopped fitting long ago. No longer will you be at the mercy of an infomercial because you'll know exactly what to do in order to look the way you want.

Now that we've laid out our goals, let's go and learn about how you can reach yours.

THE WEIGHT LOSS OBSESSION

Have you noticed how many people are obsessed with losing weight? It is truly unbelievable how this obsession can play into all other aspects of our lives. When we feel fat and out of shape, it can bring on very strong feelings of insecurity and depression. Is it hard for you to believe that not looking good can go hand in hand with not feeling good about yourself? I think not! I respect someone who might not be in the best shape but still feels very confident about himself and how he looks and feels. However, I do see that the majority of people who are out of shape are very unhappy about their appearance, and this usually transfers into most aspects of their lives.

There is increasing evidence that the American fixation with diet and weight loss is hazardous. Concerns about weight many times lead to obsessions about diet and weight control, dysfunctional lifestyles, abnormally high patterns of exercise, disordered eating patterns, metabolic depression and inadequate nutrition. Study after study has proven the ineffectiveness of dieting. Many of these studies were done on the commercial weight loss industry, including the companies who promote "losing weight." There exists a misconception that losing "weight" is the best way to feel and look good, which weight-loss companies would love you to believe. What exactly does losing weight entail? Losing weight in the traditional sense includes losing muscle, bone density, water and even organ tissue. Don't think for a second that these vital components of your body aren't being cannibalized upon during the losing "weight" stages. Is this healthy? Certainly not! But the diet and weight-loss industry will have you believe it is. Could this be a reason why people are not optimally healthy and even worse, are becoming sick? Indeed it is.

Conventional weight loss programs focus on caloric reduction, often without providing proper nutrition. These programs are not concerned with how you feel, exercise, or the reasons why you are losing weight. Reducing your caloric intake to a point where you burn many more calories than you are consuming is fine. But without exercise to help build and sustain lean muscle tissue, your body will be forced to cannibalize itself. Commercial weight loss programs can help you lose "weight," but along with that, there is a good chance that you'll also feel terrible, weaken your immune system risking sickness as a result, and in most cases gain all of your weight back plus more. In contrast, exercising will build muscle which in turn will help neutralize your fat loss. Your body will keep what you need for healthy maintenance, and burn off the rest for energy expenditures. In addition, the nutrients that you consume must be in balanced ratios that provide sufficient protein, carbohydrate and fat intake for optimal health. Do you think that these diet companies provide you with all of this? Their end result might cause you to lose weight, but not the kind you want to lose.

First we ask you to stop obsessing about your body weight. Instead, focus on bodily measurements, fat composition and the way that you look in the mirror. Why? Because weight cannot give you a true indication of how much fat you are carrying. Remember,

body weight is a combination of the weight of all of your bone structure, organs, muscles, water and fat. Therefore, if you lose five pounds in one week, how can you be assured that those five pounds were from fat? Think about it. It could have been two pounds of muscle, two pounds of water and one pound of fat. If this is the case, you are now in a worse situation than you were before the five-pound loss. Why? Because your metabolism will end up being slower and you will have lost body shape (muscle increases your metabolism and also gives shape to your body). This is why crash diets don't work. They cause you to lose mostly muscle and water, while simultaneously creating fat storage. These diets trick the body into thinking that it is starving. When the body thinks this is the case, it begins storing fat for future use and eating away at valuable muscle. So while you may achieve your ideal weight, you'll look very different than you envisioned.

Therefore, in order to achieve the look that you desire, forget about reaching your so-called ideal body weight. Humans are made up of simply too many varying frames and sizes, making it impossible to determine universal weight standards. Such a thing just isn't realistic (at least not since the 1960's). Just follow the guidelines prescribed in the Nutrition chapter and let the fat calipers, tape measure and the mirror tell you when you have arrived at your destination.

A BOOK DESIGNED ONLY FOR MEN

Men generally have different goals than women. While most women are more concerned with a slim and toned figure—more specifically one with toned and cellulite-free legs, a defined midsection, and toned arms—most guys want bulging biceps, a powerful chest, ripped thighs and a powerful back in

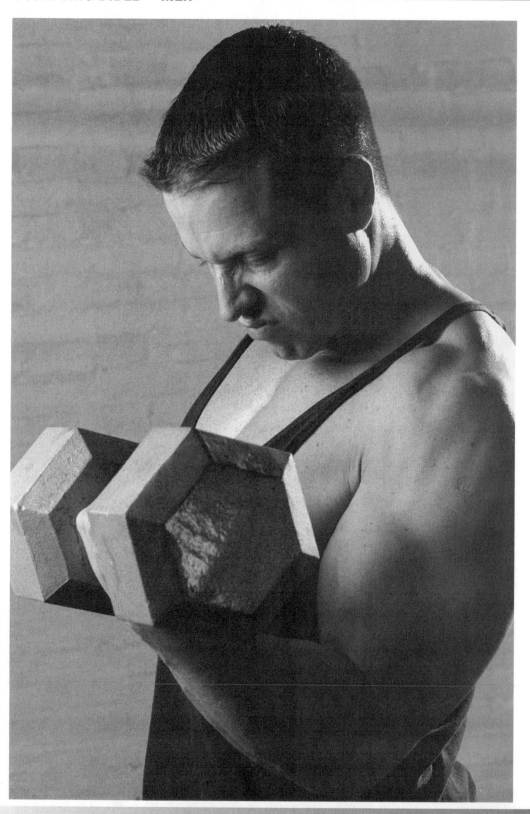

addition to losing the perfect amount of fat necessary to enable people to see a six pack on their midsection. Therefore, by taking this into consideration, we have created a program that will give you just that.

THE 14-DAY BODY SCULPTING WORKOUT

The 14-Day Body Sculpting Workout is a system that takes a safe and holistic approach to fat loss and muscle toning that enables you to reach your goals in the minimum amount of time. What is so unique about 14 days? Fourteen days is typically the amount of time that it takes us humans to get used to a new habit. Also, 14 days is the amount of time that it takes the body to start getting used to a new training and nutrition scheme. Now, while it is good for us to get used to a new habit (like waking up early in the morning to work out), it is not good for the body to get used to our workout and nutrition program. The reason for that is because once the body adjusts to your workout routine and your current intake of calories, results will cease to come! So in other words, while you will still be working out in earnest and dieting, your body will remain at the same body fat percentage and your muscles will not change any further. This is why after you start a new exercise and nutrition program, you stop getting results after a few weeks.

Why does this happen? The reason for this is because the body likes to remain in a state of homeostasis (balance). In other words, our bodies like to remain the same way that they currently are. So when you start reducing calories in order to lose fat, your body goes ahead and starts losing fat. That is until it reduces its metabolism so that fat loss comes to a standstill. You see, our pre-historic ancestors sometimes would go through periods of famine and only the fat that their bodies had

would keep them alive. Because of this, the body adapted to conserve energy (in the form of fat) in order to always be prepared for periods of low food consumption.

Now, what about muscle? Same thing here. When you start a weight training program, muscle mass comes quickly. However after a period of time of using the same routine the body learns to stay at the same fitness level. It does this in order to conserve energy as the more muscle you have, the more calories you burn. Not a good thing for our pre-historic ancestors to burn a lot of calories when no food was available. Therefore, the body is always attempting to get by with as little muscle as possible.

The 14-Day Body Sculpting Workout can help solve these problems? This exercise system:

> Changes the parameters (sets, reps, rest in between sets) of weight training routines every 14 days in a logical and manner to ensure maximum workout efficiency (more on this later).

> Adjusts the duration of cardiovascular activities every 14 days.

> Varies caloric intake every 14 days.

In addition to the above, we also include mind and visualization techniques that enable you to get the most out of your workouts. Add to that the Zone-Tone, a technique that dramatically increases the mind-to-muscle connection, plus award winning exercise descriptions and you can see why the 14 Day Body Sculpting Workout is designed to help you succeed and reach your goals!

MORE ON THE 14-DAY BODY SCULPTING WORKOUT

You may have been wondering how a 14-Day Body Sculpting Workout can exist, right? Let's get one thing straight right now. Fourteen days isn't enough time to digest a pasta dinner! Well, maybe we're exaggerating just a bit. However, all programs and/or supplements that promise you a get fit quick fix are just too good to be true and potentially dangerous to your health. We at Custom Physiques, Inc. have created the most dynamic and simple system for creating lean muscle tissue and eliminating unwanted body-fat, for good! We do not believe in starvation diets or long, exhaustive workouts in order to achieve results. We believe in a healthy, systematic and scientific approach to fitness, offering a complete fat loss/muscle-building program providing fast and consistent results. Fast Results? Yes, you heard it right! Did you think we were just going to leave the "14 day" part out? No way! Although it is physically impossible for you to completely change your body shape within 14 days (unless you have a referral to a good plastic surgeon!), you can still make some very repectable changes—to your physical body and your whole self—within that time frame. This book contains the finest fat loss and muscle building information available. How can we be so confident? We realized that we would have to take a different approach to fitness in order to make this program work best. Our strategy was to combine our own breakthrough knowledge with some of the traditional methods of fitness and health, to create the most thorough and complete fitness program ever produced. What you get is a complete and balanced approach to losing fat, building muscle and sculpting the body of your dreams.

We are about to introduce you to a new fitness training philosophy widely accepted by athletes ranging from the Olympic elite to weekend warriors and college athletes. It is called periodization training, which is defined as "a training regimen done a specific way for a specific period of time and then modified and done a different way for a specific period of time." What would be the significance of changing a fitness routine from time to time? Have you ever started a weight training routine, hoping to lose some fat while simultaneously putting on some muscle and found that it was much easier to do so in the very beginning? Do you remember how motivated you were at first and how easy it was to make immediate progress? What happened next? All of a sudden you stopped gaining muscle, you still had those last five pounds of fat attached to your body and because of that, you probably lost your motivation and desire to train. You hit a plateau and no matter how hard you trained or how much you dieted, you just couldn't make any more progress, right? What happened? Your body simply adapted! That's right, your body in an attempt to neutralize and protect your system from further breakdown (tearing down muscle and losing fat), suddenly stopped responding to the catalyst (resistance training and diet).

Periodization training prevents this adaptation. It helps to avoid plateaus, thus increasing and continually creating results. This version of the 14-Day Body Sculpting Workout was completely designed for the man whose goal is to create a more muscular and lean physique. Up until now, you have probably tried every fitness routine, gadget and/or supplement under the sun and still not reached your goals. Well don't lose hope! You will discover shortly just how powerful this program truly is.

We want to help the average guy attain his goal of sculpting a lean and muscular physique. We quickly realized that this would require certain criteria within the traditional periodization program to be customized. We knew that key components of the traditional periodization model such as sports specific training would not be necessary since the program would not be used for sports conditioning. At the same time, we realized that there had to be many specialized additions to help customize the program according to our male readers' objectives. Our main objective is to provide a direct plan of action for expediting the development of the ideal male physique (a lean and muscular body). We balanced this unique and complete revolutionary training program with the nutrition plan and a healthy mind-set method. The 14-Day Body Sculpting Workout's mind/muscle approach will help you to realize your potential!

We cannot, and will not, promise unachievable results. Unrealistic promises can both sabotage your motivation to get in shape and, even worse, jeopardize your health. Companies that make such far-fetched claims are not concerned with your well being. They only care about what they can get from you—your money. We, on the other hand, are concerned about your health. We are here to help you receive amazing results, and to explain exactly what you should do to become and stay fit and healthy forever.

Both of us have been in situations where our health and self-esteems were in jeopardy. I (James) can remember when I was 14 years old. I was very heavy and very depressed. One day while watching television, I was drawn to a commercial advertisement for a new type of diet pill called the grapefruit diet. The ad guaranteed tremendous results within a very short time period. I was young and vulnerable to such claims. I also felt desperate and immediately decided, without conducting any type of research on the company or product, to rob my piggy bank. That very same day, I sent them my money through the mail. Do you see where this is leading? I received those pills, no questions asked! They had no concern for my health, my age, or my overall well being. I took those pills and luckily, I didn't die. I see kids and adults all the time who make very similar mistakes. They have been struggling for some time, listening to claims that promise instant and miraculous changes to their physical

appearance. Do these companies ever stop to think that some people are so frustrated they are blinded by the wonderful claims and left playing Russian roulette with their lives? Do these companies realize that a good portion of these frustrated people happen to be young kids, who from being abused and ridiculed about their physical appearance, become even more frustrated and are even more willing to take any product promising to change their appearance? These kids most likely will not stop to think about the major health implications involved with taking some of these potentially life threatening products. Although there are some great companies out there, who pride themselves on creating safety for their customers, many have very little or no concern for their customers. They fulfill any order they receive, without screening or qualifying one person. We would never and could never hurt or deceive anyone. We have both come from painful childhoods and can both empathize completely with anyone who has a weight problem or any problem that relates to the body and can affect one's self-esteem. Either too heavy or too thin, we have both been through each scenario and because of that, our primary goal is to help anyone who needs or could benefit from our guidance and support. From now on, your new motto must be, "If the product or business has even a trace of uncertainty, move on!" If you don't learn to follow this motto, you will either get taken for your money and/or jeopardize your own health.

Our 14-Day Body Sculpting Workout contains only the safest, top-notch health and fitness information and techniques you need to become fit and healthy. Our program takes into account the importance of physical and mental health, and how they must be combined, in order to reach the pinnacle of good health and fitness. Our program was derived from our over 20-year combined knowledge base of health, fitness and nutrition. What we can do for you in 14 days is to totally supply you with everything you need to reach and surpass your weight loss goals. In two weeks not only will you know exactly what to do, you will actually begin to see remarkable results in a very short time. Even more exciting is the fact that the results you make during that very short time period will be permanent (provided you stick to the program) and only the beginning of your body sculpting success. Our one-

of-a-kind program integrates the body and mind, offering you a completely fit body. A body that looks and feels great! Finally, we are most excited to let you know that this will be the last weight reduction and fitness book or program that you will ever need to buy. If your goal is to lose weight and get in amazing shape, welcome to results country: This is the place where you'll find both and then some! So now it's time to get excited, as you begin the 14-Day Body Sculpting Workout, for the body of your dreams. Enjoy!

Part 1

The Foundations of Physical Perfection

Chapter 1
Common Myths & Misconceptions

1

THE BODY
SCULPTING
BIBLE
FOR MEN

In this chapter we will cover several topics that are a forum for confusion in the fitness industry.

COMMON MYTHS DEBUNKED

Myth #1: In order to gain muscle and lose fat you need to exercise for hours every day. This myth couldn't be any further from the truth. The truth of the matter is that after one hour of intense weight training your levels of testosterone (the hormone that promotes increased muscle mass and reduces fat) levels drop. Because of this, if you continue to weight train past an hour, your levels of cortisol (the hormone that destroys muscle and promotes the storage of body fat) rise, while your testosterone drops even further. This leaves you in a chemical state that encourages body fat accumulation and loss of muscle. To put it simply, more work is not necessarily better!

Myth #2: Weight training makes you stiff. If you perform all exercises through their full range of motion, your flexibility will increase. For example, exercises like flys, stiff-legged deadlifts, dumbbell presses, chin-ups, and calf raises are all exercises that greatly stretch the muscle in the bottom range of the movement. All exercises performed with a full range of motion will provide better flexibility. In training teams like the States Karate Team, we have seen firsthand this principle rejected and now accepted. It was only about eight years ago that a high percentage of elite athletes believed that weight training would make a person slow and stiff. After many top athletes finally decided to implement a weight-training regimen, they immediately noticed they were becoming stronger, quicker and more flexible than they previously had been. Therefore, by performing these exercises correctly and through a full range of motion, you will notice that your stretching capabilities will increase.

Myth #3: If you stop weight training your muscles turn into fat. This is like saying that gold can turn into brass. Muscle and fat are two totally different types of tissue. What happens many times is that when people decide to go off their weight training programs they start losing muscle due to inactivity (use it or lose it) and they usually drop the diet as well. Therefore bad eating habits, combined with the fact that metabolism is lower due to inactivity and lower degrees of muscle mass, give the impression that the subject's muscle is being turned into fat—while in reality what is happening is that muscle is being lost and fat is being accumulated.

Myth #4: Weight training turns fat into muscle. More alchemy. The way a body transformation occurs is by gaining muscle through weight training and losing fat simultaneously through aerobics and diet. Again, muscle and fat are very different types of tissue. We cannot turn one into the other.

Myth #5: As long as you exercise you can eat anything you want. How we wish this were true! However, this could not be further from the truth. Our individual metabolism determines how many calories we burn at rest and while we exercise. If we eat more calories than we burn on a consistent basis, our bodies will accumulate these extra calories as fat regardless of the amount of exercise that we do. This myth may have been created by people with such high metabolic rates (lucky them) that no matter how much they eat or what they eat, they never meet or exceed the amount of calories that they burn in one day. Therefore, their weight either remains stable or goes down.

UNNECESSARY GADGETS

Let's talk about all of the exercise contraptions we see on TV. Why do we need to pay over $80 to perform an abdominal crunch? The abdominal crunch is perhaps the most simple exercise there is to target the abdominal muscles. Do we need a machine to help us do it? We think not!

Ads for such gadgets promise abs in minutes a day. But did you ever read the fine print on the TV screen? It usually reads that the statements are true as long as you combine the exercise with a sensible diet—which brings us to the next point. You do not need to enslave yourself everyday to hours of abdominal work (only 5 to 10 minutes of ab work is sufficient). What really brings out the definition in your midsection is a sensible nutritional program combined with weight training and aerobic exercise. Together, these components burn fat in order for definition to appear. The abdominal work only builds the muscle covered by the fat. Besides, there is no way in which you can reduce the fat in only one section (spot reduction) without reducing it in the rest of your body.

Once again why would you need to purchase an ab machine? To make the exercise simple? Exercise isn't supposed to be easy! If you expect it to be, you can expect little or no results. Unless you are recovering from a back injury and are not yet strong enough to do a crunch by yourself, save your hard earned dollars for more meaningful things. All you need to perform an abdominal crunch is the right knowledge describing how to execute the exercise correctly and the floor.

If one of the reasons for purchasing an ab machine includes the benefit of avoiding neck strain, this is also not a good reason. If you don't know what you are doing, you can strain your neck with or without the machine.

FAT BURNING CREAMS

We have all seen commercials that promise to eliminate fat by rubbing the latest cream discovered in some exotic locale. At Custom Physiques Inc. we have talked with many guys who have used such products with no results. Good luck finding any real scientific research on the subject that proves these products work. Again, save your hard earned money.

The only thing that eliminates fat from your body is a systematic approach to eliminating it through the nutritional practices we describe along with a training routine that is designed to tone and eliminate body fat from all angles. That is the only way that the battle of the bulge can be won. Don't let anybody mislead you.

WEIGHT LOSS CLINICS

Why pay others every month to tell you what to do when you are fully capable of figuring it yourself after reading this book? We have seen what most weight loss clinics offer and we are not impressed! Not only do you pay an unbelievable fee (sometimes on a monthly basis) to get a diet that may not be as efficient as it could be (most of these programs are low protein diets); some require you to buy special foods (provided by them, of course, on top of the initial fees they charge.) Others charge you by the pounds you lose. Hey, what a concept! You do the work and you get to pay someone else for your success!

DRUGS FOR WEIGHT LOSS

If what you want is health and permanent weight loss, don't touch any kind of weight loss drugs. Most are very dangerous (remember Phen-Fen?) and can cause serious side effects such as heart problems and possibly death. Besides, once you stop using them you begin

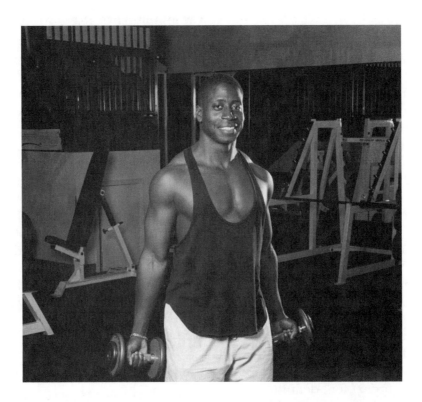

to gain all of the weight back. So what's the use? People criticize bodybuilders for using steroids and everybody preaches how dangerous they are. Well, using weight loss drugs (and this includes those formulas that claim to be natural but contain caffeine and ephedrine) is exactly the same thing! There is nothing different here; it's using dangerous drugs in order to achieve a pleasing cosmetic effect.

When Phen-Fen came out people flocked to their doctors to get a prescription. Unfortunately, many were given the drug despite the fact that research indicated that this drug combination had some serious side effects. The drug was soon pulled from the market.

The only solid and safe solution that takes the weight off permanently is the correct combination of diet, exercise and rest. Anyone who tries to convince you otherwise is full of it! Therefore, once again, save your money, but more importantly, save your health.

THE MOST COMMON & FATAL DIETERS' MISTAKE: THINKING THAT EATING LESS IS BETTER

When people think of a diet they think of pain, hunger and food deprivation. At first, most dieters reduce their food intake dramatically and see that in the first week they lose as much as 10 pounds of weight. They say: "Great! In order to lose more weight I need to eat less." After a few weeks they notice that they are not losing as fast as they had hoped. Frustrated, they start to starve themselves even more. Before we continue, let's stop right here and explain what is going on inside the body.

The first week the person will lose weight as the metabolism gets shocked by the decreased food intake. However, most of the weight lost is derived from water with only 3-4 pounds coming from fat. The second week the body, still not adjusted to the shock, continues to lose weight (though not as fast as the first week).

By the third week the body begins to take counter measures in order to adjust to the lowered caloric intake. Think about it; what do you do when your light bill goes up? You probably begin to save electricity in order to save money. The body naturally reacts just like you consciously would. When it sees that its metabolic costs are too high (in other words, losing fat because the metabolism is too high) then it decides to save energy and lowers your metabolism in an attempt to keep the fat on. Therefore, the person experiences a slow down in weight loss or just comes to a standstill. The way you save electricity is by turning energy hungry appliances off, right? The way your body saves energy is by losing muscle, because muscle is the most expensive tissue to maintain.

So by looking at the scenario above, let's see what may happen to someone (we'll call him Joe) who is determined to lose weight but does not know how to go about doing so.

As Joe notices that his weight loss comes to a sudden halt, he decides to reduce his caloric intake further. For the first few weeks this in fact works, but afterwards the weight loss comes to a standstill again. After a few cycles of the same thing, Joe continues to spiral downward. At this point most people (99 percent) just forget about the diet and start eating everything in sight. They gain back all of the weight and then some (remember it will be easier for them to gain weight now because they lowered their metabolism by using the wrong dieting practices). However, there is a very determined 1 percent of dieters who will not give up.

These people continue the cycle described above. They begin to look pale, and feel cold. They are hungry all the time but deny it. Sometimes they go without food or water for the whole day. They look at themselves in the mirror and they still see themselves fat, even though everyone tells them that they are already skinny (very skinny). They are afraid to drink water because they think water will make them gain weight. This terrible condition is called anorexia nervosa, a condition that I (Hugo) suffered from in my early teens. Despite what most people think, this condition is not one that only affects women.

People with this condition are not totally crazy in seeing themselves as fat. Even though they look very skinny in clothes, if you take their fat percentage you will probably see that it is around 20-30 percent. The reason for this is because the body has shed plenty of its muscle tissue, but maintained as much fat as possible. Initially, anorexics usually create a goal consisting of a completely different physique, one that is toned, hard and firm. In the hopes of attaining this physique they continue on their downward spiral. However, they never seem to achieve what they originally hoped for, so they decide that the best thing to do is eat fewer calories. See how the cycle is created?

The only cure for conditions such as this one is education. We remember that when we used to be overweight everybody used to tease us, poke fun at us and tell us to "just stop eating!" People treated us as if we were diseased. Therefore, we decided to take action and started doing what people told us to: We stopped eating!

However, the only solution for losing weight (fat) and keeping it off while at the same time building a lean and hard physique is eating the correct combinations of food, along with doing weight training and aerobic exercise. So please, never fall into the trap of thinking that eating less will get you good results!

BULIMIA

Another eating disorder, bulimia (characterized by bingeing and purging) is somewhat of a difficult subject for me (James) to write about because I personally battled with it for a period of time in my life. When I was young, my physique was the last thing on my mind. I did not care about how I looked or what I ate. Being served seconds for lunch and dinner was not enticing for me; it was more like thirds and fourths that got my attention. My mother, who is a registered nurse and an amazing one at that, was not aware of the health implications and effects that too much food would cause to my body. As a matter of fact, most health practitioners, including medical doctors, are not always aware even today, of some of the implications food can have on a person's body. As I grew older and **larger** I was forced into realization of my obesity. One day, while in Junior High School, a gym teacher pulled me aside and made me step onto the scale. I weighed about 200 pounds at age 12/13. He thought that his way of revealing my weight problem to me was a productive one. He was wrong! The only thing he did was embarrass and anger me.

From that point on, I began to gain more and more weight until finally I was at my all time high of 255 pounds. I was fat and depressed and had no idea what to do about my problem. I resorted to weight loss pills and liquid diets, which only frustrated me more. My sister, who was also quite heavy, began suddenly to lose weight. I was shocked at how she shed pounds of weight, yet didn't diet or exercise. It was odd, but I started to notice that her once beautiful olive complexion began turning pale. In addition, I would constantly see her falling into a deep depression accompanied by anxiety. I, like most people with eating disorders, paid no attention to the terrible things that she was going through. I just wanted to know how the heck she was losing that weight. Well I found out!

Staying up late and having good ears made it obvious. I could hear her throwing up in the bathroom and knew that this was the way she was losing weight. While I was afraid to try

such a harsh thing, I went ahead and tried it. At first, I hurt the back of my throat by gagging. I then tried other ways to purge myself, all of which were ways of causing a gag reflex. That was when my terrible eating disorder began. In the beginning I lost some weight and actually felt good because I could eat junk food while getting the results I wanted. That was until I noticed some odd behavior in myself, such as an obsessive need to exercise and ongoing bouts of low self-esteem. I felt like my self-worth required that I be skinny. I continued until one day, while living with my parents, I heard my sister scream from the bathroom. I ran upstairs and tried to open the door, but it was locked! I screamed for my sister to unlock the door, but she didn't. I had to break open the door and found my sister on the floor naked, lying in a pool of water. She had fallen out of the shower due to her body becoming weakened by the abuse of bulimia. She was purple and looked as if she was having a seizure. I screamed to my mother and she immediately called the police. It was discovered that she had developed seven bleeding ulcers, among many other problems that were all the side effects of bulimia. I was never so scared in my life as when I saw what my sister had done to herself and realized that I was on the same path.

Since that time, my sister and I have both stopped abusing our bodies and have educated ourselves about eating disorders. With strong will and persistence, we conquered this eating disorder and I must say that my sister has become a beautifully strong and confident woman. We discovered through reading and from our personal dealings, that even though a person with any eating disorder may look happy and cheerful, that person is often depressed, lonely, ashamed and empty inside. Friends of bulimics may describe them as people who are competent and fun to be with. But underneath all of that, where they hide their guilty secrets, they are actually hurting badly. They may feel unworthy and have great difficulty talking about their feelings. These feelings are often accompanied with anxiety, depression, self-doubt, and deeply buried anger.

So you see, bulimia is a very dangerous eating disorder that will never meet your expectations of acquiring a great looking physique. Bulimia is a disease and one that needs to be taken care of with the help of someone knowledgeable. Please remember that bingeing and purging is not the way to get in or stay in shape. *If you feel that you may have this terrible disease, please seek professional counseling.*

LOW CARB/HIGH PROTEIN/HIGH FAT DIETS

Low carb (less than 50 or even 30 grams a day), high protein, high fat diets might at first work. The reason? After the initial adaptation period of two weeks, in the absence of carbohydrates, the body has no choice but to go into a state of ketosis (carbohydrate deprivation) and start burning fats for fuel (this is assuming that more than 50% of your calories are coming from good essential fatty acids like olive oil and flaxseed oil). Basically, your body shifts its carbohydrate metabolism into an exclusively fat burning metabolism. Now, like any diet, the same basic principles apply. Even though you will be burning fats exclusively this does not mean that you will be able to eat everything and anything without getting fat. Remember if you take in more calories than what you burn, you will get fat.

We have tried such diets for as long as a year at a time. In our opinion the following are the drawbacks:

- As you can imagine, if you are only allowed 30-50 grams of carbohydrates a day, your life will not be very tasty. You will only be limited to a small selection of foods.

- Even though at the beginning you lose incredible amounts of weight, it is mostly water weight. We also did not find a big difference between losing fat in a low carb diet and losing fat on a moderate carbohydrate diet. Both diets provide similar benefits.

- While on a low carbohydrate diet, the muscles feel flat (shrink in size) due to the fact that the glycogen (the carbohydrates that are stored inside the muscle cell and make the muscles look firm) gets depleted. On a moderate carbohydrate diet, your muscles always feel firm and tight.

- We experienced joint pains after the ninth month on the diet. We were drinking two gallons of water a day so lack of fluids was not the problem. We wonder if it was the lack of carbs that caused the fluid in the joints to diminish but this is mere speculation. Once we switched back to a moderate carb diet, the joint pains disappeared.

- You have to pay close attention to your cholesterol levels and to nutritional deficiencies caused by the lack of variety in the diet.

- In order to get all the good fats in the diet, we had to take them in liquid form; not very tasty.

In our opinion, even though this type of diet might work, we don't believe it can be maintained for a lifetime. If you feel like trying it, then please remember to pay close attention to cholesterol levels and nutritional deficiencies. However, we believe that to get in shape the best approach is a more balanced one.

STEROIDS; THE GOOD, THE BAD AND THE UGLY

The purpose of this section is not to teach you how to use steroids, nor to endorse or disapprove of their use. We mainly write this section as an informational tool for those who are curious about the subject and also to eliminate certain misconceptions that surround these drugs. Our goal is to write an unbiased report that gives the objective information regarding what these drugs are and what they can and cannot do. This is based on research and information that we have gathered from others that have used them. We cannot share any personal experiences in using them as we have never touched them.

WHAT ARE THEY?

Anabolic steroids are a synthetic copy of the hormone testosterone. They have been the subject of much debate and misinformation over the last few decades. Athletes, especially bodybuilders, may feel lured towards them as these drugs do increase muscle size, strength, and stamina. One of the biggest misunderstandings is that people say that if you take steroids they will kill you. The first thing we need to understand is that steroids are drugs. All drugs when misused and abused have the potential to kill; not only steroids. Even Tylenol and Aspirin can cause serious problems if you take them in large quantities. Another misconception out there is that they are easily accessible and that there is only one type of steroid. As far as accessibility, the truth is that they are illegal substances so their accessibility will be through the black market (good luck as far as quality). In addition, if you get caught with them in your possession you may face up to five years in a federal prison. On the issue of variety, there are many different types of steroids out there. There are liquid steroids that you inject and there are pills that you take orally. The injectable kind are generally more anabolic in nature and less damaging to organs like the liver. The oral versions are more androgenic in nature and cause more side effects than injectables, as they have to be processed by the liver. Different steroids have different properties; some build muscle mass while others increase strength or decrease fat. As their properties vary, so do their side effects; stronger steroids (especially oral) have more side effects.

THE GOOD

Steroids do increase size and strength. In fact, they do so very significantly. We once conducted a small informal research study in which we compared the results of a bodybuilder on steroids with those of a natural bodybuilder (in this study, we participated as the natural participants in order to ensure that all training and nutrition aspects were dialed in). The enhanced bodybuilders gained strength and muscle mass at an accelerated rate (as much as 50-60 pound strength gain per week on the big basic exercises and around a 40 pound muscle mass gain in 6 weeks. Note: The subjects were stacking four different types of testosterone in large dosages and their diet, training and rest were dialed in). Needless to say, 12 weeks later one of them entered a local contest and won hands down.

In addition to potentially massive gains in strength and muscle mass steroids also seem to provide you with more energy and aggressiveness, things that can be conducive to good workouts.

THE BAD

Because steroids can provide many beneficial effects it is no surprise that they cause psychological dependence. If you have been taking steroids for the past eight weeks, assuming you are on a good diet and using a thorough training routine, chances are that you have gotten very big (muscular) and strong very quickly. One of the feelings people on steroids usually claim to have after approximately eight weeks of use is an "unstoppable" feeling. When you begin to taper off them, you might still experience these "highs," but will it last? Once you completely stop using them and after cessation of use, you very likely will notice that you are not getting good pumps, your strength will start to diminish regardless of your best effort and your muscle mass will begin to atrophy (shrink!). Add to that for the first few weeks after cessation of use, you will most likely experience bouts of depression, due to low testosterone levels.

It is no wonder that a large number of steroid users never stop taking these drugs.

THE UGLY

Assuming that you knew what you were doing while you were using steroids (i.e. getting consistent blood work done while using them, using a mild steroid, ensuring that the dosage taken was not overboard, making sure you tapered off before complete cessation of use and taking a break from their use every 12 weeks or so), chances are that you will still experience depression after use, plus loss of strength and muscle mass. You will most likely notice a period of low natural testosterone production (in addition to other side effects that may be encountered during their use, such as higher blood pressure and higher cholesterol levels). We have gathered research claiming that administering mild steroids with proper use can aid in maintaining a percentage of muscle mass gains. However, we have seldom heard of a steroid user who maintained much of anything after steroid use (except for some side effects), which puts the validity of those claims in question. Based on our observations, steroid use will ultimately provide more losses than it will gains.

If you are careless with your steroid use (i.e. using high potency steroids causing many side effects and/or abusing the dosage you administer, etc.) then not only can the side effects be numerous during the period of use, but you also will also experience terrible side effects after cessation of use. Again, the degree of side effects you personally experience is directly proportional to the dosage and type of the steroid you use. It is also dependent on the genetic propensity of the subject which will ultimately determine the side effects they receive. Therefore, it would be impossible for us, or anyone else, to precisely predict what type and how many side effects a user might encounter during a period of steroid use. However, below we have listed a few of the side effects users have experienced from steroid abuse:

1) Increased liver function.
2) Depletion of testosterone levels.
3) Increase in cholesterol levels and blood pressure (Not beneficial for good cardiovascular health).
4) Altered thyroid function.
5) Migraine headaches.
6) Nose bleeds.
7) Muscle cramps.
8) Development of breast-like tissue in men (Gynecomastia).
9) Insulin insensitivity (Even though the steroid Deca Durabolin has been known to improve the insulin metabolism).

10) Androgenic side effects such as thinning hair, enlarged prostate, oily skin, water retention, increased body hair, physical aggressiveness etc.

11) Stunted growth in teenagers.

12) Oral steroid specific side effects: In addition to the above, the oral steroids also tend to cause nausea, diarrhea, constipation, and vomiting.

13) May accelerate the growth of tumors.

CONCLUSION

Having said all of the above, we would now like to include our two cents worth (here comes the subjective part of this section). We are not going to just come out and say: "Don't use steroids; they kill," as by now you could probably make an educated conclusion. There are many drugs available both by prescription and over the counter, that in our opinion are just as dangerous as steroids. However, it seems to us that using steroids only provides fleeting glory and a temporary solution to the challenge of acquiring muscle mass. At best, you might get bigger for a while, but how much is that worth to you? Is it worth risking your health and/or jail time in order to gain a few pounds of muscle? If you happen to get these drugs from the black market, how can you be assured that the quality of them is good? How will you know for sure exactly what you are putting into your body? Will it be pure or contain contaminants? If you are using an injectable steroid, how can you be sure that you will be able to consistently inject it correctly, without causing an infection on the site of injection or possibly pinching a nerve? Finally, how can you be sure that you don't have a propensity to develop cancer and that by using steroids, you won't assist in speeding up the process? These are all things that you should think about if there is ever a time when you are tempted to use these drugs. Building your body into a beautiful work of art should start with a lifetime commitment, one that is practiced eagerly, day in and day out with the utmost persistence. There should never be any shortcuts when it comes to creating your ideal physique. Relatively hard work combined with smart training and a sound nutrition system will take you exactly where you want to go.

Chapter 2
The Power of the Mind

Powerful Methods for Achieving Success

2

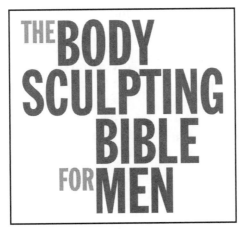

THINGS DON'T ALWAYS HAVE TO BE AS COMPLICATED AS THEY MIGHT SEEM; NOT WHEN YOU LEARN HOW TO STRATEGICALLY AVOID COMPLICATIONS.

What you have in your hands right now is a straightforward and logical formula that we have broken down and simplified, making the information easy to comprehend and follow. This manual gives you the most effective sure-fire plan to attain a better looking body, in the shortest amount of time humanly and naturally possible.

The subtitle of this book is "Featuring the 14-Day Body Sculpting Workout" because if you follow the guidelines that we present, you will start to notice amazing changes in your body within a couple of weeks. Please understand that this is not a magic program. We are not claiming that your body will miraculously change overnight. However, by applying the enclosed methods to your lifestyle, along with applying yourself to the program, you will achieve results and then "magic" may just be the word you'll use to describe our program. Often, people who have seen us train ask, "How do you make such noticeable physique changes with such a short workout?" That's just it! That's the underlying formula, the key to your success. Remember more is not necessarily better and in the case of this book, definitely not. If you understand how the body works, you will be successful in the shortest time possible. We live in a fast paced world, where time is a precious asset. We don't have the time to spend long hours in the gym—even a short time in the gym can be a major commitment. Having extra time can greatly enhance your life, allowing you to do some of the things you've otherwise neglected. A basic, yet scientific approach to fitness training is what's needed, and is exactly what you're about to discover with the 14-Day Body Sculpting Workout!

DIFFERENT ROUTINES: SOME WORK, MOST DON'T!

"What kind of workout routine should I choose?" This is probably one of the most frequently asked questions when it comes to exercise. With so many different routines and so-called "guru philosophies" out there it would surprise us if only a few people were confused about this issue. Deciding what program to choose can be extremely difficult. Even professional trainers and elite athletes frequently have problems choosing a quality program. There are many different programs—some good, some bad, some terrible. The fact of the matter is that some of these programs may in fact work, if you dedicate yourself to them. That is the key word, "dedication." The dedication we mean is the dedication of devoting yourself and your time (remember you are not in the gym to waste time!) to something, to get as much out of it as is humanly possible. To do this, you must define exactly what your training objectives are before and during a fitness session. Without this mindset, you will undeniably fail to achieve optimum results. You must realize that when you're not prepared you cannot expect to receive the maximum response from your actions, and therefore you will not see results. You must know what tools (exercise and technique) to use and what to expect at each workout session in order to receive your desired effect (more muscle tone and less fat). You also must make sure that your response or reactions to the stimulus are as accurate as you expected them to be.

The basic guidelines and training principles of your fitness program must always be based on information that is backed by scientific fact. This particular routine is the exact routine that all of our male clients at Custom Physiques Inc. have followed and they have received phenomenal results. Please understand that the routine alone is not enough to make your dream body appear. You must follow the proper training methods and initial preparation techniques included in this book to help make the program work optimally. Using correct exercise form alone is very important for steady results. If you follow the proper, often neglected, training techniques, form and principles we describe, this program can be the program that changes your life forever! We do realize that there are currently several schools of thought concerning the best types of weight reduction and body sculpting workouts. We also realize that most of these so-called, state of the art programs lack useful information and will not live up to their claimed benefits.

The 14-Day Body Sculpting Workout is based only on concepts that truly work. We include some traditional principles, which supply the building blocks of all reputable fitness programs, as well as new and exciting principles and techniques that are considered breakthroughs in the field.

EXPECTATIONS AND DESIRE; EXPECT AND YOU SHALL RECEIVE

Where would we be without our expectations? It happens to be a driving force in our ability to plan effectively. If you want to be a success—in the gym or in the office—you must set goals for yourself. But setting goals is not enough. In order to reach those goals as smoothly and as quickly as possible, you must think about what it is that you expect to receive.

When you begin the 14-Day Body Sculpting Workout, expect optimal results. Expect to receive what you bought this book for. By

doing this you are creating a positive mind-set, a vital component of this program. Once you commit yourself to anything, do not question its power or validity (unless of course it's dangerous). Instead, dedicate yourself to it until you've accomplished your objective. Many of the fitness programs available today would work somewhat if the above mindset were followed. Now imagine what you will accomplish by creating a positive mind-set with this program. You are almost ready to begin your journey to success. Why a journey? Because all of the following techniques can be applied to all aspects of your life! Now let's move on to our first powerful tool for success.

MIND SCULPTING: VISUALIZATION AND MENTAL IMAGERY (THINK AND BECOME!)

These techniques can provide great accomplishment of your fitness goals, and virtually all aspects of your soon to be (if not already) amazing life!

Before you can sculpt your body into a piece of art you must first sculpt your mind into a powerful tool. How would you like to guarantee success and accelerate your results exponentially? This next portion of the 14-Day Body Sculpting Workout addresses a very powerful technique that is virtually non existent in the fitness realm. It happens to be one of the most pragmatic life changing methods used in the history of human potential. The special tool we speak of is known as visualization or mental imagery. In the next few minutes you are going to learn how to develop and use some fantastic capabilities that lie dormant within each of us. They will allow you to perform remarkable feats that you would have never believed possible. You can realize your dreams if you focus your thoughts on what you want for long enough.

You may ask how such influences occur. The mind has an all-powerful control over matter:

Your body is a prime example of such. Do you know that medical doctors consider many illnesses psychosomatic, that is, caused or provoked in part by the patient's own thoughts? Even diseases such as cancer may have psychosomatic origins, since the power of our minds over our bodies is so strong.

Right now, you are going to learn how to cultivate a talent for visualization that you already possess within you. This power is more or less developed from one person to the next. But, with the right training anyone can achieve excellent results. Just as exercise develops the muscles, the appropriate physical and mental training will make you a master of visualization. The balance of body and mind exercise is too often neglected, but is the key to astonishing success!

There are three conditions that you must have in balance for optimum results. The first is **desire.** How can you expect to obtain anything, if you don't want it badly enough? Desire is that fire you feel in your belly when you so badly want something, creating the **drive** and **determination** to achieve. The stronger your desire, and the more sustained it is, the more certainty you add to reaching your goals quickly. In order for your desires to become powerful, you have to feed them with the intense fire of your will and imagination. How? By thinking about them on a daily basis and imagining that your goal has already come true.

By doing this, you will be in the optimum mental state to make your goal a reality. Your mind will attract the events that are capable of producing the results you seek.

The next component in the model is **discipline,** the essential condition for all personal development and accomplishment. Without this component, you cannot expect to achieve or accomplish great things. In order to become fulfilled, your mind needs discipline. How can

you expect to accomplish or receive anything at all if you're not able to fix your attention on the goal you have set out to achieve? Do you really want to lose weight and get into great shape? The disciplined individual possesses a strong and confident attraction to his goals. The disciplined person succeeds where most fail, and always ends by conquering the obstacles blocking his path. The person who could care less about creating discipline constantly falls prey to failure. No matter how many other great qualities this person may possess, for this person success is the exception rather than the rule. Most of the time he ends up where he is by chance; certainly not by choice. So how do you learn and practice discipline? By tirelessly repeating exactly what it is you want to achieve in your life. You must constantly remind yourself of what it is you are out to achieve (more muscle? less fat? better tone? more definition?) from your fitness plan. The same can be done for other aspects of your life. Discipline your mind, apply the principles we've outlined here, and you will realize wonderful results.

The last of the components in the model is **action**! Even if you possess desire and discipline, without action you will never obtain what you want. Combining **action** with **desire** and **discipline** creates the three musketeers of achievement. Many people have great ideas, foolproof plans and creative knowledge, yet everything falls apart for them. Why? Because they never act or they never act persistently enough. *The difference between a person who knows and one who succeeds resides in the individual's ability to act.*

Everything that you read in this book is the fruit of experience born of practice. If you apply the techniques and principles that we have discussed and you put action into the equation, you will meet your goals with astonishing success. Many people wrongly believe

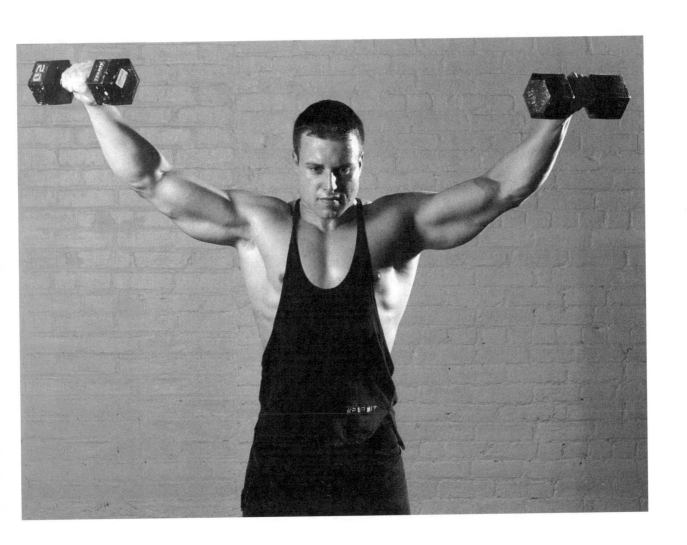

APPLYING THE VISUALIZATION TECHNIQUE: AN INTRODUCTION TO SELF-HYPNOSIS FOR UNPRECEDENTED RESULTS

Before beginning a visualization session, you must be fully rested. As the body needs adequate rest for exercise and activity, so does the mind for concentration and focus. Have you ever noticed that when you are tired you can't keep your concentration and things don't seem to work? When you feel like this, don't continue trying; take a nap! This allows for optimum concentration, the most important subcomponent of the visualization technique.

Try to set aside a time for practicing the method. It will only take about 15 minutes a day to put the technique into action. But without a set time, procrastination can and will set in, making it impossible to find the time needed. By setting a specified time each day (i.e. right before sleep or upon morning rising) you will condition your mind to be ready and effective every day at the same time. Also, try not to eat prior to the session because it will divert your needed energy (just as you should not eat prior to a workout for circulatory and digestive reasons.) Be enthusiastic about your sessions too. Take pleasure in knowing that you are on your way to your personal best physique.

When practicing visualization you don't have to force it like exercise. Take it easy and relax! We are not doing bodybuilding exercise, yet the results achieved will blow your mind! The more relaxed you are, the clearer your image will be, thus allowing for more powerful results.

The first step in practicing visualization is to become entirely relaxed and calm. If you have already had some practice with relaxation or self-hypnosis techniques, you should be able to relax very quickly. We will assume that you have no experience with relaxation techniques.

First, direct of your energies towards obtaining a state of very deep physical and mental relaxation. Your mind-set will be that you feel remarkably calm and relaxed. We will now cover in detail a self-hypnosis session to rid your body of tensions and help to relax you completely.

Stretch out comfortably on your favorite recliner or lay in your bed. Next, concentrate on one single point: either directly in front of you or above you (the ceiling, for example). Begin by saying the following sentences either out loud or to yourself, consciously focusing on feeling the physical effects they produce on you.

> "My mind is fully concentrating on my focal point and the harder I concentrate on this point the more my mind and body are relaxed." (Note: Take as much time as necessary to feel the intended effect of total relaxation.)

> "My eyes are getting more tired and my eyelids are getting heavier with every passing second." (Focus on your heavy eyelids as you fall deeper into your desired state).

> "I want to close my eyes, and I close my eyes."

> "I feel totally calm and relaxed. My body is getting heavier and heavier, sinking into my bed (or seat). I can feel myself so, so relaxed. My eyes are now completely closed and I am so, so relaxed, yet focused on my body." (Do not fall asleep; you are relaxed,

not sleepy!) "I will now begin to consciously relax my body." (Always begin with your feet, focusing first on your toes and moving body part by body part up towards your head. Proceed as outlined below with the following suggestions.)

"I am concentrating all of my attention onto my feet, which are growing heavier and becoming so, so relaxed." (You may start to feel a tingling sensation as if very slight pins and needles were in your feet and toes.)

"A very comfortable and warm feeling is vibrating throughout my entire body."

"I will now focus on my legs, which are beginning to sink deeply into themselves." (Concentrate on this feeling but do not force it. This should be fun, not work! When you practice regularly, you will automatically fall into the desired state quickly.)

"My stomach is now beginning to feel very heavy, sinking deeper and deeper into itself." (Allow for relaxed and easy breathing to occur. As you progress and move on to each body part, simply allow that part to lazily relax while you concentrate on the amazing feelings of relaxing your body. What you are doing right now may very well change your life forever!)

"My hands and fingers are growing heavier and heavier. They are totally relaxed."

"My chest is now sinking deeper and deeper into itself. With each breath I fall deeper and deeper into relaxation. I feel so, so calm and relaxed; I feel a warm vibration throughout my whole body."

"My neck is growing heavy and feels so relaxed as I allow it to sink deeply into itself. My head is relaxing more and more. I feel no pressure, only the heaviness allowing my head to sink deeply into itself. All of my thoughts are calming and relaxed. I feel as if I am in a dream floating."

"In this mind state, every thought that I wish to focus on is so powerful, so very powerful that nothing can stop it from becoming reality, whatever the obstacles in my way." (Repeat this last sentence mentally three times).

Now form a mental image of exactly what it is that you want to achieve (a totally ripped or defined physique, more muscle, smaller dress size, entering and winning a competition, losing ten pounds of fat, gaining ten pounds of muscle,) visualizing the object or goal towards which your message will be transmitted. The image must be as vivid and real as possible. Keep it in your mind's eye for about ten to fifteen minutes, without going over fifteen minutes.

Think about your message strongly. Do this for ten to fifteen minutes depending on the state of relaxation you have achieved. If you start getting tired or tense, stop, rest and begin in a few minutes. Think about your message by concentrating all of your attention on it. The more you are absorbed by it, the stronger the effect, thereby creating better success. The more the message is present in your mind during the session, the greater your success. Act with conviction that your message will come true.

Don't forget that everything you believe will come true. This is the universal rule. Act with desire, discipline and faith to achieve. These actions cannot fail to produce the desired results.

What you have just read and experienced is a technique that really does work. We passionately believe in the power of the technique for attaining an abundance of success and achievement in your life. You can apply this powerful visualization technique to any and all aspects of your life. It is universal. Enjoy!

You may find relaxation and visualization foreign; you may not be comfortable with it. However, in order to change your life and make your desires reality, you must be willing to do what may initially be uncomfortable or different. The visualization technique can change your life, but only if you open your mind to change. Don't be afraid of change. You have the power to open up and accept new challenges. Are you capable of letting go and willing to try new things? *If you want to dramatically change your physique and create a more exciting life for yourself, then take some chances, move out of your comfort zone and open your mind and life to new possibilities.* These mind powering techniques are not commonplace or commercialized. Most teachers, whether it be fitness or academics, are afraid to teach what is not ordinarily taught. They are scared to cross the threshold of beliefs in fear that they will be the first to teach a method and possibly fail. We are not afraid to teach you our methods because we are confident that what we teach works: it has worked for us and thousands of others as well. We are simply revealing what may be the single most powerful life changing tool in existence. Open your mind and begin to make changes where you never thought possible.

that anything that doesn't fit their way of thinking must be false. Unfortunately for them, these people limit themselves by thinking that they are always correct. They never put their own beliefs into question. Whatever you do, never allow yourself to become this type of person. Always question others and follow your own instincts; but most importantly, **act as often as possible**!

THE ZONE-TONE CONCEPT

One of your goals is to get in great shape as quickly as possible, right? If you don't know already, you will soon discover that the mind-to-muscle connection coupled with proper exercise technique and form are crucial if you want to stimulate the necessary muscle fibers needed to create a dynamite physique. While this may seem obvious and common sense, strangely enough, most people neglect the mental aspect behind exercise execution. It is not unusual to go to a gym and see people that are just "going through the motions;" in other words, moving a weight from point A to point B with little stimulation being directed towards the working muscles.

In this section you will learn another powerful technique that will immediately provide astonishing performance and enhanced results to your physique by teaching you how to develop your mind-to-muscle connection!

We have named this very unique concept the "Zone-Tone" method. It is the art of mentally zoning in and pre-isolating specific muscles just before an exercise is to be executed while at the same time maintaining that zone throughout the execution of the movement. This wonderful technique is very easy to grasp and will deliver enormous benefits to your fitness program. Combining proper form and technique (something that you will learn in the

upcoming sections) with the Zone-Tone method will help you reach all of your fitness goals much faster than with conventional practices. You will discover that the level of isolation and stimulation that you feel within your muscles will increase tenfold any time you perform an exercise using this method.

There are several reasons why people fail to create a successful mind-to-muscle connection:

- Lack of human body anatomy knowledge combined with a lack of information available showing how to successfully create a mind-to-muscle connection.

- Misinformation on the part of our teachers or books regarding exercise execution. In other words, people getting the wrong kinds of advice.

- Most people have a difficult time with change—they become accustomed to doing the same thing day-in and day-out. As a result, they refuse to change the way in which they conduct their exercises.

- Lifting gargantuan weights without any concern for proper exercise form and technique, in order to simply satisfy our ego.

Of all of these possibilities, perhaps the biggest reason why people are not familiar with the mind-to-muscle connection is the lack of information available on the subject, coupled with a lack of knowledge on basic anatomy. If we asked you where your biceps were, would you be able to point to their exact location on your body? Are you aware that there are actually two biceps muscles, hence the prefix "bi"? Now, the next question is, if we asked you to flex your biceps muscle, could you do it effectively? How about the hamstring muscles located behind your thigh. Could you make that muscle contract really hard? Let's talk triceps; those three relatively small muscles located on the back of the upper arms. If we asked you to squeeze those muscles hard so that they tensed up intensely, could you do so immediately? The answers to these simple questions will soon lead to perhaps the most profound, beneficial and eye opening mental exercise technique the fitness industry has ever experienced. (**Note:** Please do not feel bad if you do not know where these muscles are located. Our job is to teach you where they are and how to use them. **Appendix J** is a simple anatomical chart that contains the location of each muscle group.)

Now, when you're getting ready to do an exercise, do you ever stop to think about exactly what muscles you are about to train? Some of you will say yes and mean it. Some of you will say yes and not tell the whole truth. Most of you will say NO! This is the amazing reality that we are dealing with. We must admit to you that we truly love this fact. We love it of course, because we are the ones who will teach the world how to correctly and effectively transform their physiques ten times quicker than they previously could have, by simply mastering this method. We love it even more due to the fact that because most of you have never learned how to activate the mind-to-muscle connection while performing an exercise means that you all have a tremendous window of opportunity for major improvements to be made to your physique!

The key to improving the mind-to-muscle connection is to become attuned to our bodies and enhance this connection to the fullest potential, before and throughout the exercise movement. This means knowing precisely what muscles you are targeting before you start the exercise and moving the muscle from its fully extended position to its fully contracted position (full range of motion), while consciously focusing on feeling the muscles (and only the

intended muscles) contract and extend throughout the entire movement. Carelessly going through the motions of exercise is a complete waste of time and a great way to get nowhere very quickly.

SO HOW DO WE USE THE ZONE-TONE METHOD?

While the Zone-Tone concept might seem like a difficult technique to learn, it is not! You might think that you won't be able to do it effectively or learn to use it quickly, but we will show you that in fact you can! We have taught it successfully to many others and now we will do the same for you.

There are only two simple steps to the Zone-Tone method:

Step#1: Focus and zone in on the individual muscle/s you intend to train before you begin the exercise. Before each and every set of an exercise, focus and zone in on the individual muscle(s) you intend to train (for this, knowledge of where each muscle is located is crucial; look at the anatomical chart in Appendix J.) Tense and flex the muscle to be trained as hard as comfortably possible before you even start to execute the exercise. This way you will be sending a message to that muscle, preparing it by completely isolating it even before the exercise begins. By doing so you have successfully created a mind-to-muscle connection.

Step#2: Maintain your mind-to-muscle connection during the execution of the exercise. Throughout the execution of the exercise, deliberately feel the muscle elongate (stretch) and contract, as you move from point A to point B (the full range of movement for a particular exercise). What we really want you to do while you are performing the exercise is to (flex) the muscle as hard as you can in the same way you did on step 1, but with the

THE 10 COMMANDMENTS OF BODY SCULPTING PERFECTION

Commandment #1: Believe in Yourself! If not, you won't be able to achieve your desired results!

Commandment #2: Write down your goals. How can you get somewhere if you don't know where you are heading?

Commandment #3: Set new goals every six weeks. After six weeks, compare your results against what you had in your original goals.

Commandment #4: Place a calendar on your fridge. Mark a back slash on the days that you followed your diet without cheating. Make a forward slash on the days that you trained. If you trained and followed a good diet on a given day, you should have an X marked on that day.

Commandment #5: Place a picture of how you currently look somewhere that you will be able to see on a daily basis. This picture should provide you with additional motivation to follow this program.

Commandment #6: Take pictures of yourself every 4 weeks and place them on the refrigerator next to your "before" picture. That way, whenever you have a craving and go to the refrigerator you will remember the reason that you are doing this and also get motivated by seeing the progress that you are achieving.

Commandment #7: Write down the reasons why you are following this program and put them on your refrigerator. Same benefit as item 6.

Commandment #8: Keep your house free from any foods that are not good for your program. Only on Sundays can you bring these foods in the house.

Commandment #9: Remember to prepare all your meals the day before. If you bring your food with you to work, you are less likely to give in to your temptations..

Commandment #10: Remember that only you control what goes in your mouth. Food does not control you!

exception that now you have a weight in your hand. This is crucial as it is of no benefit to activate the muscles before the exercise begins if the mind-to-muscle connection is lost as the movement starts. Most people waste their time by exercising without thinking about what they're doing. They exercise on a physical plane rather than on both the mental and physical planes. This is fine if you are content with average results, but who really wants to be average? On the other hand, if you want to compound your efforts exponentially and undeniably create the body you've always dreamed about having, then you must effectively develop the mind-to-muscle connection that we have been describing to you here.

When you effectively call out to a muscle and prepare it for the oncoming set you create a mind-to-muscle connection. By keeping this connection throughout the execution of the exercise, that one set will produce the results of five sets! Do you realize what this can mean for you? If you implement these principles into your training regimen, you can create unbelievably toned and incredibly defined muscles in half the time! Imagine then the type of results that you will get by combining the Zone-Tone method with the 14-Day Body Sculpting Workout and the exercise execution techniques that are later presented in this book. We guarantee that by combining all of these concepts, you will achieve the most astounding and unbelievable physical transformation in the minimum amount of time.

FURTHER ENHANCING ZONE-TONE'S EFFECT

How would you like to multiply the effects of the Zone-Tone method? Here is a way to compound your efforts with little or no additional time expenditure.

Remember what you did during your meditation and visualization sessions as you focused on relaxing each and every muscle in your body starting with the feet? Well, at this time you have an invaluable opportunity to implement the Zone-Tone method.

IMPLEMENTATION

Starting with the feet, as you begin to relax and focus upon your toes, slightly wiggle your toes and concentrate on feeling even the slightest movement in each individual toe.

You might actually feel a little strange tingling sensation as you may have never stopped to pay attention to the feeling of these individual parts of your body. You might wonder why we would waste time focusing on the feet first, right? We want to do this so that you become completely familiar and in sync with each and every part of your body. This will eventually give you the ability to isolate any muscle you desire at will. It is very important to remember and focus upon each and every part of your body without neglecting any specific part! As you move on from the feet towards your knees and up, zone in on every body part along the way. Now here's where it can get tricky so pay attention. Simply focusing on the individual muscles of the body is not enough. When you simply think about them you cannot truly get a feel for how they feel when they are in action. To help you hone in and experience the feel for each of these muscles you should do the following:

- As you get to each individual body part, stop and contract the muscle as best as you know how. Do this three to five times and then relax.

- Remember the exact area where you felt that muscle contract and now focus all of your attention and energy on relaxing that same area. You are giving yourself an amazing ability to become in complete control of your entire superficial muscular system and will have the opportunity to call upon their action for maximum muscular efficiency.

Here is yet another technique you should use to further enhance the effects of the Zone-Tone method:

- After you complete each set of an exercise, stand in the mirror and contract the muscles that you were exercising as hard as you can and hold for a count of 3-5 seconds. What will this do for you? It will help you to create a stronger mind-to-muscle connection and help you to accurately identify and call upon those individual muscles during exercise.

We can't tell you enough how important it is to practice the Zone-Tone method both when you're working out and at rest. As with anything, the more you practice the Zone-Tone method the quicker and more powerful the method will become. Soon you will realize first-hand the astonishing results gained from this powerful concept. Good luck!

LIFE'S DILEMMAS, SIMPLE SOLUTIONS; SOME PEOPLE MAKE EXCUSES, OTHERS FIND SOLUTIONS

In life we are bound to face adversity or dilemmas at one time or another. When this happens the key is to not freeze up. This is the problem many people have. Instead of doing something to help solve their problems, they dwell upon them, feel sorry for themselves, and let the problems overtake them. In order to become successful at anything in life, instead of accepting adversity, **combat it!** Instead of feeling sorry for yourself or just dealing with the problem, **find solutions for the problem!** By finding solutions, you never

give in to failure. You never admit defeat, and therefore are never defeated. It is only when you admit and give in to failure that you become a failure. The most successful people in the world have learned this philosophy and adapt it to their lives on a daily basis. Finding a solution to a problem is not as hard as it seems. You must use your imagination in order to achieve solutions. You must be willing to do what most people are not willing to do. Namely, you must create solutions by using your talents. Brainstorming is one such talent, in which you write down any and all ideas to help solve your problem. This might be a quick fix, such as changing an exercise or the sequence of exercises you perform during an exercise session. It might be a long-term solution, such as the one you discovered by applying these new principles into your life. The goal here is to be creative and "think outside the box!" Whatever solution or strategy you choose to apply, just make sure it is realistic and of sound knowledge.

In the next section, you will learn why it is important for you to understand that your subconscious mind cannot tell the difference between a real experience and one that you imagine. Can you imagine the benefits associated with that!

THE BLUEPRINT FOR A PERFECT BODY

The method below is an extremely powerful tool that can help you accomplish any of your goals (both in and outside the gym). If you're as skeptical as we once were, try to let go of your inhibitions and open up your mind to endless possibilities. People don't realize how incredibly happy and successful they can be with just this one technique. So we hope that you make good use of it.

The conscious mind has the ability to conjure up fantastic dreamlike images of the things you most desire. However, it is the sub-conscious mind (that feeds from the informa-tion you program into it with your conscious mind) that can turn your imagined visions into realities. Your subconscious mind reacts not only to what is actually true, but also to what you imagine. Your subconscious mind will store emotional fantasies or dreams as reality. For instance, if you see yourself with a per-fectly lean and muscular body, and truly believe this is possible, you are programming your subconscious mind with your imagination to bring this dream into reality.

Creating a mental blueprint of your dream body with your conscious mind is the first step. But when you program these mental blueprints into your subconscious mind believ-ing that you can have them, or better yet, believing that you already have them, your subconscious mind will go to work for you to devise the methods that will make your fantasy come true. Creating a desired mental picture or blueprint in your mind provides the intellect with a profound principle. The value in creat-ing mental pictures is enormous in that it gives the mind a constructive course of action to follow. It can and will help guide and moti-vate the practitioner into doing what is neces-sary in order to succeed. How would you like to see yourself in the next two months? Would you like to lose five inches around your waist? Would you like to gain five pounds of lean muscle for an unbelievably attractive body? Would you like to make a complete metamor-phosis of your body shape? If you said yes to any one of these, or perhaps have other desires that you'd like to attain, it is to your utmost advantage to incorporate the "mental blue-prints" method into your life. This same tech-nique can be applied to any other aspect of your life as well.

In order to receive the best results from your visualizations, you must learn to create the

proper mindset. Creation of the proper mindset method is not a "think positive and everything will be great" type of method. This powerful weapon is fantastic for wiping out any negative thoughts, helping to keep you on the right track to success! Combining the right attitude with the proper training (visualization and blueprint imaging) is the surest way to quickly reach your goals.

The attitudes you project during your daily life can play a significant role in determining future occurrences. In other words, consciously paying attention to your thoughts and changing them if necessary into positive thoughts is important for an optimal life and the creation of wonderful things.

Too many people have no faith in them-selves. They have no belief that they can actu-ally create better things or a better life for themselves. If you believe in yourself, have strong desires and act upon them with faith, desire and diligence, then that dream body, that beautiful house, that nice car, that won-derful life can all be yours. Your subconscious mind will react automatically to give you whatever you program into it, either real or imagined. (Haven't you noticed that when we have a bad dream, the body reacts as if it were a reality; heart rate, adrenaline and blood pressure go up. The mind cannot distinguish the difference!) Your subconscious mind will not take the trouble to work for you unless you truly believe what you program into it. You must visualize or see yourself the way you want to look. It is also highly important that while transmitting your intended message to your subconscious mind you do so in the spirit that you already possess your dream body (or possess whatever it might be that you wish for). Have confidence in yourself and your goals, making sure that nothing or no one gets in the way of reaching them. You must realize, unfortunately, that many people will not want you to reach your objectives, not always intentionally, but sometimes because of insecurities of their own. You must learn to stay clear of these people and, even more, to stay strong in your convictions. If someone says that you cannot do or achieve certain things, use that negative energy as a way to fuel your determination in order to get you exactly where you want to be! By doing this, you will conquer any and all obstacles in your way and reach your goals.

Realize that you must use these mental images in order to fuel your determination to help commit yourself and do what you have to do in order to achieve success (e.g.: train, eat right and rest). Just believing that it is possible to reach your goals is just not enough; we need to take **action** in order to get there.

In conclusion, the secret to achieving success is to program what you want into your subconscious mind by believing in yourself and seeing yourself as you would ultimately like to look or live. Such mental programming will then motivate you to set a plan (in this case a sound workout and nutrition program), follow through with the plan, and persevere. By programming yourself for success, everything you desire can and will be yours.

THE MANY BENEFITS OF EXERCISE AND CORRECT EATING: YOU WILL GET MUCH MORE THAN YOU HOPED FOR!

Exercise provides many benefits:

Benefit #1: Increased energy levels. When you exercise and eat right your energy levels go through the roof as the body is working at peak efficiency. This is due to the fact that the correct combination of diet and exercise produces a hormonal environment that leads to increased energy, fat loss and increased muscle tone.

Benefit #2: Increased mental focus. Did you know that exercise actually boosts brainpower? That's right; in fact, the latest research indicates that exercise can help keep the brain sharp well into old age, and might prevent many diseases, such as Alzheimer's disease, along with other mental disorders that accompany aging. If the brain is able to operate in peak condition, imagine the improvements that could be attained with business, decision-making, brainstorming, and every aspect of your life. Think of your brain as you do a muscle. If you train it, it will become conditioned. You train your brain by introducing new challenges like reading new information or learning a new skill such as the many you are now learning while reading this book.

Benefit #3: Increased self-esteem. When you begin feeling good about the way you look, your self-esteem automatically goes up. This leads to self-confidence, empowering you with feelings of control, stability and a wonderful ability to make critical decisions under pressure.

Benefit #4: Increased sense of control over your life. Once you are able to change the way you look and feel with exercise, you'll notice that you can change anything else that you want in life by using the same basic principles that allowed you to make such a transformation possible (Desire, Discipline, & Action). No longer will you be afraid of setting a goal and not meeting it. If you are able to change yourself, you can change anything else that surrounds you (within reason of course).

Benefit #5: Reduced chances of heart attack. By exercising and dieting you lower your cholesterol, blood pressure and stress levels, greatly reducing your risk of having a heart attack.

Benefit #6: Reduced chances of osteoporosis. Correct exercise and diet practices increase bone density, reducing your risk of osteoporosis.

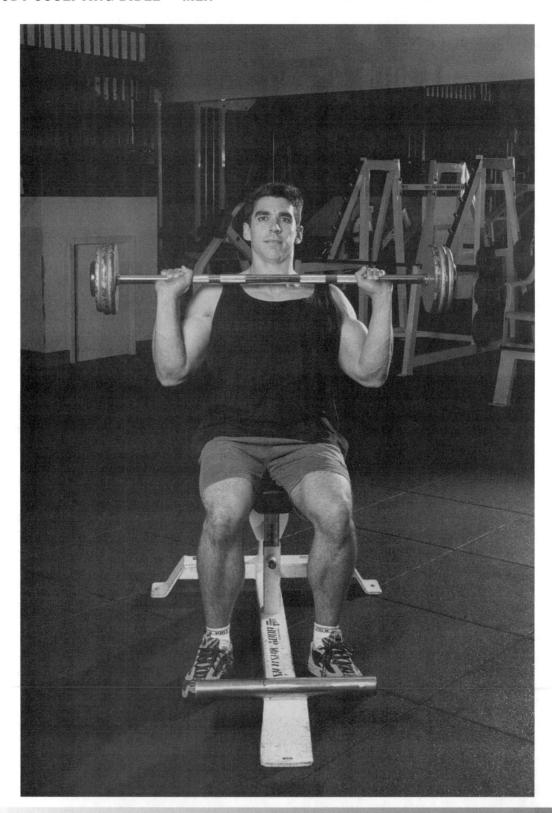

Benefit #7: Increased strength and stamina. Naturally, exercise provides you with more strength and stamina that inevitably become extremely useful in your daily activities.

Benefit #8: Less depression. Exercise increases your production of endorphins (hormones that make us feel good and happy). Due to increased endorphin production, your chances of getting depressed are greatly reduced. Did you know that it was recently documented in medical journals that the benefits of exercise are equal to that of the benefits associated with taking anti-depressant medication? That's correct, you can receive some of the same calming and balancing effects that prescription medication provides, just by engaging in daily exercise and all without the potential side effects! (The information presented here *does not* suggest that you stop taking your prescribed anti-depressant medication or any medication prescribed by your medical doctor. It is simply a positive addition to the many benefits associated with exercise).

Benefit #9: Exercise helps control stress level. Note that with exercise, worries dissolve while mood rises. Say you had a bad day—the traffic was horrendous, the boss was in a foul mood, the phones wouldn't stop ringing, and you were late for an important meeting. Could you imagine going to bed with all of that accumulated stress you've got? Most people must deal with the stresses surrounding them, but think back to how we discussed finding solutions rather than letting dilemmas get the best of us. Adding therapy such as exercising right after work (for those of you that like late afternoon training sessions) is a great natural therapy that helps to release your stress, while secreting those powerful endorphin hormones that make us feel amazing.

TURN OFF THE STRESS LIGHT!

If you feel like you are stressed and it's time to go to sleep, try this technique to help you "turn off the stress light." When you lay down in bed, first relax your entire body by quickly going through the steps of the relaxation technique you learned in **"Applying the Visualization Technique,"** beginning on page 26.

Once you feel physically relaxed, mentally picture a light bulb in your head that is turned on. You can clearly see in your mind's eye how bright that light is. You can also see in your mind's eye the on/off switch for the light, located on the wall right next to the light. Now imagine that this light represents your mind which is currently turned on and so very bright. The bright light indicates that there is a lot of activity going on, and, the more stress you are dealing with, the brighter the light will be.

Now, think strongly about how that light switch located on the wall can either be left in the turned on position or simply turned off. If you leave the light turned on, the activity will continue. Maybe you need to think and put some things into perspective.

If you wish to rest, putting all of your thoughts and stresses to sleep, then you need to turn that light off! That's right, in your mind's eye, put your finger on that light switch and get ready to turn off that light, which represents all of the thoughts in your mind.

You must focus strongly on making the connection between that light and your mind's activity. When you turn that switch to the off position, the bright light you see in your mind's eye will automatically go black, and with it will cease all activity in your mind.

Just relax and let yourself fall deep into relaxation once you see the darkness. At first, you might need to repeat the turning off the light switch process a few times before you feel the strong connection take place, but don't force it! The whole process will eventually become quite natural and you will soon find the technique nothing short of remarkable. In fact we've been using the technique for several years now and it never fails to work wonders for helping us fall asleep quickly. The next day you'll be refreshed and ready to tackle anything the day throws at you. One of the most important things to avoid while training is sleep deprivation. You can read about the side effects associated with this problem on page 96.

THE FORMULA FOR SUCCESS

Since we are engineers it is hard for us to write a book containing no formulas. Consider the following formula for success in changing your appearance; it is based on determination.

$$S = D \times (T+N+R)$$

S is the success that you achieve in your program, D is your determination to succeed, T is your training, N is your nutritional program, and R stands for rest.

Each component in the formula above can only have two values. A value of 1 is given to a component if it is followed completely. A value of 0 is given to any component that is not followed or just followed halfway. Therefore, if every single component is followed, you get a maximum value of 3. In this case you would get the fastest results possible from your program. If you stop following one of the components inside of the parenthesis then you get a lesser value and sub-optimal results. However if you don't have any determination, you get a value of 0, your whole program fails, and you don't get any results. The reason? *Determination is by far the most important factor in determining the amount of success you will achieve in your Body Sculpting Workout.*

After examining the formula above, it is easy to see why just purchasing a sophisticated gadget or a couple of magic pills at the health food store is not going to cut it. In order to achieve permanent weight loss all of the factors described above have to be present and in perfect harmony. Follow one but not the other and your success will be negatively affected.

THE FIRST COMPONENT: DETERMINATION

Determination is the first component the formula for good reason. Of all of the four components that make up the formula this is the only one that is more important than the others. If you are not determined enough to make the sacrifices necessary to get in shape, then nothing is going to happen. You can have all the knowledge that we have on how to get in superb shape, but if you don't apply it then all you have is wasted knowledge. You need to want to change your appearance as badly as you would want to breathe if you were drowning. You also have to believe in yourself and know that you can do it. You must not doubt your ability to change. **If you have doubts, you will fail!** You will also need tunnel vision; in other words focus on your goal and no matter how much adversity you encounter stick to your plan, follow through, and get there. It is not an easy path. In a day and age where skepticism and negativity rule, roadblocks will appear (such as people telling you that you will not succeed or putting your program down). Every time you encounter a negative situation like that, use it to your own advantage. Use it to fuel your desire to achieve your goal. Don't let anybody put you down! This is important stuff. This not only applies to changing your appearance; this applies to every aspect of your life! If you set your mind to something and want that something badly enough, you can attain it, no matter what the circumstances may be. Set a goal, develop an action plan and follow through with it—no matter what happens—until you reach that goal. In this book we give you a proven plan to change the way you look. Whether you want to lose a few pounds of fat and put on 15 pounds of lean muscle or lose 100 pounds of fat and put on 5 pounds of lean muscle, we provide you with a road map on how to get there. Use your desire and put the plan to work for you.

THE OTHER COMPONENTS OF THE FORMULA FOR SUCCESS

In the next few chapters we will cover the topics of training, nutrition, and recuperation. Due to the enormous amount of information necessary to thoroughly cover these topics, we have decided to dedicate a full chapter to each one of them.

Chapter 3 covers your training plan, **Chapter 4** discusses your nutrition plan and delves into the importance of supplements and **Chapter 5** is dedicated to the often neglected components of rest and recovery.

Part 2

The Building Blocks of Body Sculpting

Chapter 3
Training

3

THE **BODY**
SCULPTING
BIBLE
FOR **MEN**

Training is the first component inside the parenthesis of the formula for success. The way you train will ultimately determine the way you look. This is how you will be able to sculpt your body into a work of art.

There are two types of training: Anaerobic exercise (e.g. weight training), which uses glycogen as its main source of fuel, and aerobic exercise (e.g. walking, bike riding, etc), which uses oxygen as its main source of fuel. We will discuss each separately and then go into detail about each type.

WEIGHT TRAINING

The anaerobic training that we will be using is weight training. Weight training is the number one way to resculpt your body. It is far superior to any other form of exercise because it is the only one that can give shape to your body and increase your metabolism permanently. This is vital since a slow metabolism is at the root of obesity. We find it ridiculous that some fitness authorities don't adhere to this simple yet very true concept. It is ludicrous how some "fitness experts" believe that aerobic exercise is the key to the perfect physique. **These "authorities" are wrong** and should educate themselves by learning the facts.

GOALS

Without goals we are dead in the water. We have nowhere to aim and nowhere to go. Therefore we need to set goals in order to achieve success.

Our body sculpting goals are going to be the following:

Gain: 10-25 pounds of muscle (or more depending on how muscular you want to look) in order to tone up and increase the metabolism.

Lose: Enough fat to get down to 10-12% body fat (or less than 10% but no less than 6% depending on how defined you would like to look).

Depending on where your physical fitness level is at this moment, it may take you longer than six weeks to achieve these goals. However, don't feel bad about that as the important thing is that you will be moving forward and you will achieve these goals very quickly by being persistent and consistent with your fitness program. Besides, remember that by doing nothing, in a year from now your body will look the same as it looks now—or worse.

Now that you know where you're headed, let's see what the characteristics of a good weight-training program are.

CHARACTERISTICS OF A GOOD WEIGHT-TRAINING PROGRAM

In order for weight training to be effective, the following rules should be followed:

Sessions should be short: 60 minutes maximum. The maximum amount of time a weight training session should last is 60 minutes. After 60 minutes the levels of muscle building and fat burning hormones (like growth hormone and testosterone) begin to drop. In addition, the glycogen (stored carbohydrates) in your system, which is the fuel that your muscles use to contract, is depleted. If you weight train more than 60 minutes you will actually be wasting your time since you will no longer have the hormones or the fuel necessary to produce muscle growth. Continue to train past 60 minutes and you will get impaired recovery, which leads to overtraining, a condition where your body does not recover from its weight training sessions. This leads to loss of strength and muscle mass.

The rest between sets should be kept to a minimum; 90 seconds or less. Keeping your rest time in between sets and exercises to a minimum not only allows you to perform a prodigious amount of work within the 60-minute weight training window, but also helps improve your cardiovascular system and most importantly maximizes the output of growth hormone, a powerful fat burning/muscle building hormone. Also, this rest interval promotes a muscle voluminizing effect in which water goes inside the muscle cells (not outside) and makes the muscles look more firm and toned. Do not confuse this with water retention outside of the muscle cells, which is what makes us look puffy and fat.

Sets of each exercise should consist of 8-15 repetitions. There are many reasons for this. First and foremost, it has been shown that it is within this range that growth hormone output is maximized. As we already know, this is a good thing since this hormone does exactly what we are looking for (it increases muscle and decreases body fat). In addition, since you are performing so many repetitions, you get a great pump (blood rushing into the muscle) that provides nutrients to nourish muscle cells and helps them recover and rebuild faster. Finally, performing 8-15 repetitions reduces the possibility of injury dramatically since you will need to use a weight that you can control in order to perform the prescribed amount of reps. (Note: This rule does not apply to the calves and abdominals as these muscles usually respond better to higher repetition ranges, in the order of 15-25 reps).

Training must be progressive. Progression means one more repetition than the last time the exercise was performed or a little bit more weight if you are able to do more than 15 repetitions for a particular exercise. It is important to understand that you will not be able to increase weight or the number of repetitions every session. However, progression comes in many forms; like performing more work within the 60-minute period. The overall goal of a training routine is to ensure progression over a period of time to bring about continuous improvements in muscle tone and definition.

Training must be varied. This principle is vital to ensure continuous gains in strength and muscle tone as well as to prevent boredom. Variation does not necessarily mean changing all of the exercises in your program. Variation can occur in the form of using different techniques to stimulate the muscle, changing repetition and set parameters, and even changing the rest in between sets. It can also be something as simple as changing the width of your grip placement on the bar to help isolate specific muscles. As you will soon see, the 14-Day Body Sculpting Workout makes full use of this principle, since every two weeks your routine changes, providing you the variation that your body needs to keep moving forward.

Training must consist primarily of free weight basic exercises. Only free weight basic exercises provide the fast results you are looking for because they recruit the most muscle while you are performing them. Besides, the body is designed to be in a three dimensional universe. Whenever you use a machine you limit your body to a two-dimensional universe and consequently you limit the amount of muscle fibers that are going to do work. Not all machines are bad, however. Some definitely have a place in our weight-training program because they allow us to isolate the muscle in a way that no free weights would allow us to do. However, our program should be mostly based on barbells, dumbbells and exercises where the body moves through space (such as the dip, the pull-up and the squat). The best exercises for each body part are the following:

BACK

BASIC EXERCISES

Wide-grip pull-ups (or pull-downs if unable to perform pull-ups) to front, close-grip chin-ups (or close-grip pull-downs if unable to perform chin-ups) with palms facing your body, chin-ups with a neutral grip with palms facing each other (or close-grip pull-downs with a V-Bar if unable to perform neutral grip chins), one-arm rows, two-arm rows, pullovers, bent over barbell rows.

ISOLATION EXERCISES

Stiff-arm pull-downs, low-pulley rows

CHEST

BASIC EXERCISES

Incline bench press (and its dumbbell version), flat bench press (and its dumbbell version), chest dips, and push-ups

ISOLATION EXERCISES

Chest flys (incline and flat versions), incline cable crossovers

THIGHS AND BUTTOCKS

BASIC EXERCISES

Barbell squats (and dumbbell version), ballet squats (and dumbbell version), lunges, leg press

ISOLATION EXERCISES

Leg extensions

HAMSTRINGS

BASIC EXERCISES

Stiff-legged deadlifts (and its dumbbell version), leg press (feet high on the platform), lunges (how far you extend your leg when you do this exercise determines which leg muscle is activated the most. The farther away from the torso that you extend your leg, the more you hit the hamstrings).

ISOLATION EXERCISES

Lying leg curls, standing leg curls, seated leg curls

SHOULDERS

BASIC EXERCISES

Military press (and dumbbell version), upright rows (and dumbbell version)

ISOLATION EXERCISES

Lateral raises, bent-over lateral raises, rear-delt machine

BICEPS

BASIC EXERCISES

Dumbbell curls, barbell and dumbbell

preacher curls, incline dumbbell curls, hammer curls, and reverse curls, E-Z bar curls

ISOLATION EXERCISES

Concentration curls

TRICEPS

BASIC EXERCISES

Barbell and dumbbell lying triceps extensions, barbell and dumbbell overhead triceps extensions, triceps dips, close-grip bench press (and dumbbell version)

ISOLATION EXERCISES

Triceps pushdown, triceps kickbacks

CALVES

(Note: For calves and abdominals there is really no distinction between basic and isolation exercises)

Standing, seated, and donkey calf raises, calf raises on leg press machine, one legged or two legged calf raises with dumbbells

ABDOMINALS

Crunches, leg raises, and knee-ins, trunk curl and crunch, V-ups

AEROBIC TRAINING

Aerobic training such as walking or running on a treadmill is a good way to accelerate the fat burning process (as long as it is not overdone and is used only in addition to a good weight training program). It should never be used as a substitute for weight training since it does not permanently increase your metabolism and does not have the ability to reshape your body.

In order for aerobic exercise to be effective, it needs to be performed within the fat burning zone. The fat burning zone is the zone at which you are doing just the right amount of work to burn fat. Your pulse (how fast your heart is beating per minute) determines this zone. It is important to remain in this zone for a certain period of time. If you work harder or longer than what the formula recommends, it will quickly lead to exhaustion which will prevent you from continuing to perform the activity for a prolonged period of time. On the other hand, too low of an effort will not prompt your body to start its fat burning mechanisms.

To determine your fat-burning zone, use the following formula:

Fat burning zone = (220-Your Age) x (.75)

For example, a 20-year-old man would need to reach a pulse in the neighborhood of 150 beats per minute in order to be in the fat burning zone. It is important to remember that this is not an absolute figure, but an approximation. As long as you stay within 10 beats of the number that the formula provides, you can rest assured that you will be burning fat.

Another important point is that in order for aerobic exercise to be an optimal fat burner it needs to be performed at the appropriate times. There are two ideal times where aerobic exercise is most effective in burning fat. The ideal time is first thing in the morning on an empty stomach after drinking 16 to 24 ounces of water in order to prevent dehydration. Exercise performed at this time burns 300 percent more body fat than at any other time in the day because your body does not have any glycogen (stored carbohydrates) in the system to burn. Therefore, it has to go directly into the fat stores in order to get the energy necessary to complete the activity. The other time that aerobic exercise is effective would be immediately after a weight training session as your glycogen stores have already been depleted. Because of this, once you start doing your cardio, you will start burning fat as soon as you elevate your heart rate since it is the only fuel that will be available.

When aerobic exercise is not performed first thing in the morning or right after the weight training workout it takes your body approximately 20 to 30 minutes to start burning fat because that is how long it takes the body to deplete its glycogen stores and switch to a fat burning environment. Therefore, it is not as efficient to perform aerobic exercise alone at other times of the day because you would need to work out for 20-30 minutes just to get to the fat burning stage and then continue to work out for an additional 20 minutes to burn fat. This would mean a grand total of 50 minutes a day. In our opinion, aerobic exercise shouldn't be performed more than 6 times a week for 40 minutes maximum each session, in order to avoid losing muscle mass. Remember that more is not always better and this is especially true when it comes to aerobic exercise. As you will see, for this program (unless you are interested in bodybuilding competition), the most you will be doing is three sessions lasting between 20 to 40 minutes each at the most.

Good forms of aerobic exercise include riding a stationary bike, fast walking (this can be done on a treadmill), climbing on a stair step-

per, swimming, using a fitness rider or rowing machine, using any good cardio tapes like Tae-Bo, or any other form of cardiovascular activity that raises your heartbeat to the fat burning zone.

PUTTING IT ALL TOGETHER

Now we will learn how to put all this knowledge together in a workout program that will yield the results. We present three different workouts. Which one you should choose will depend on your previous training experience and your fitness goals.

The first workout (*the Break-In Routine*) is to be used by men who have never done weight training before. This program is a break-in program that will not only allow you to get in shape quickly, but will also condition you to get in the shape necessary to be able to use the 14-Day Body Sculpting Workout.

The second workout (*the 14-Day Body Sculpting Workout*) is for men who have been weight training for at least ten weeks and want to get into awesome shape (gain 10-25 pounds of muscle and reduce body fat to 10%).

The third workout (*the Advanced 14-Day Body Sculpting Workout*) is the most advanced workout to be used only by men who either have an interest in bodybuilding competition or just want to look like a bodybuilder (gain 25 pounds of muscle or more and reduce body fat to 6%). This last workout requires at least one year of weight training experience in the gym and is the most time consuming of all workouts. It will emphasize all angles of the muscle in order to produce the most stunning Body Sculpting effect. Therefore, this workout is reserved for the most serious fitness guys out there.

Before we present the 14-Day Body Sculpting Workout, let's discuss a few terms that you need to understand in order to execute the routine.

Repetitions or reps: The amount of times that you perform an exercise. For instance, imagine you are performing a bench press. You pick up the bar, lower it, pause and lift it up. That action of executing the movement for one time counts as one repetition. If you perform that same movement a second time, then that is your second repetition and so on and so forth.

Sets: A set is a collection of repetitions that culminates in the muscle reaching muscular failure. Muscular failure is the point at which, due to a buildup of lactic acid in the muscle, it becomes impossible to perform another repetition with good form.

Rest Interval: The amount of time you rest between sets. For instance, a rest interval of 60 seconds means that after you finish your first set, you will remain idle for 60 seconds before going on to the next set.

Now that we have discussed these important terms, let's discuss the main techniques that make the 14-Day Body Sculpting Workout so effective.

Modified Compound Supersets: In a modified compound set, you pair exercises, usually for opposing muscle groups or for opposing muscle movements (e.g. push vs. pull). First you perform one exercise, rest the recommended amount of seconds and then perform the second exercise (for instance, first do biceps, then do triceps). Then rest the prescribed amount of time again and go back to the first exercise. A modified superset for Dumbbell Curls and Triceps Pushdowns in which you perform 4 sets of each exercise will look like the following:

Dumbbell Curls Rest 60 seconds	1 set of 10-12 reps
Triceps Pushdowns Rest 60 seconds	1 set of 10-12 reps
Dumbbell Curls Rest 60 seconds	1 set of 10-12 reps
Triceps Pushdowns Rest 60 seconds	1 set of 10-12 reps
Dumbbell Curls Rest 60 seconds	1 set of 10-12 reps
Triceps Pushdowns Rest 60 seconds	1 set of 10-12 reps
Dumbbell Curls Rest 60 seconds	1 set of 10-12 reps
Triceps Pushdowns	1 set of 10-12 reps
End of modified superset	

You will be resting a total of 2 minutes plus the amount of time that it takes you to perform the other exercise, so you actually are resting a given muscle between 2.5 and 3 minutes. Using this technique of pairing exercises in a **modified** superset fashion not only saves time and keeps the body warm, it also allows for faster recovery of the nervous system between sets. This allows you to lift heavier weights than if you just stay idle for 2-3 minutes waiting to recover. An additional benefit of this technique is that it saves time and limits rest to a maximum of 90-seconds in between sets.

Supersets: A superset is a combination of exercises performed right after each other with no rest in between. There are two ways to implement a superset. The first way is to do two exercises for the same muscle group at once (like dumbbell curls immediately followed by concentration curls). The drawback to this technique is that you will not be as strong as you usually are on the second exercise. The second and best way to superset is by pairing exercises of opposing muscle groups (antagonists) or different muscle movements such as back and chest, thighs and hamstrings, biceps and triceps, shoulders and calves, upper abs and lower abs.

When pairing antagonistic exercises, there is no drop of strength whatsoever. As a matter of fact, sometimes your strength increases because the blood in the opposite muscle group helps you perform an exercise. For instance, if you superset dumbbell curls with triceps extensions, the blood in the biceps helps you do more weight during the triceps extensions. Because of this, we will only perform supersets where opposing muscle group or opposing muscle movement exercises are paired. Supersetting not only allows you to do more work in a shorter period of time but it also increases endurance, creates an incredible pump (especially when you pair antagonistic exercises), and helps burn fat by elevating the heart rate to the fat burning zone (which also gives you cardiovascular effects). Also, because of the stress created by this technique, growth hormone levels go through the roof. Remember that this hormone is responsible for fat loss and enhanced muscle tone.

Giant Sets: Giant Sets are four exercises done one after the other with no rest in between sets. Again, there are two ways to implement this. You can either use four exercises for the same muscle group or perform two pairs of opposing muscle group exercises. For the purposes of this book whenever we do Giant Sets, we will perform two pairs of opposing or different muscle group exercises with no rest (the exception is in abdominal work in which we will alternate between lower abs and upper abs).

A Giant Set for biceps and triceps in which you perform 4 sets of each exercise looks like this:

Dumbbell Curls (No rest)	1 set of 10-12 reps
Triceps Pushdowns (No rest)	1 set of 10-12 reps
Hammer Curls (No rest)	1 set of 10-12 reps
Lying Triceps Extensions (60 second rest)	1 set of 10-12 reps
Repeat sequence 3 more times.	

Giant Sets provide you with more of the same benefits that supersets have to offer. This is the most intense and powerful technique that we will use in our 14-Day Body Sculpting Workout. We need to be cautious when using Giant Sets since they are considered an extremely intense exercise protocol. Although the human body is capable of handling great intensity and stress, you should never push it to the edge. The Giant Sets protocol is a very powerful and results oriented training method, but should be used sparingly. In our program the Giant Sets protocol will only be used for about two weeks. Have you ever heard the saying that "too much of a good medicine is bad?" This certainly applies to Giant Sets. This is really strong medicine in the fight against fat. Use it for more than two weeks and your body will no longer be able to recover; the nervous system will get burned out and will reach a state of overtraining, where your body can no longer recover from the workouts.

Now that we have discussed the three techniques that are the basis of the 14-Day Body Sculpting Workout, let's see what the routines look like.

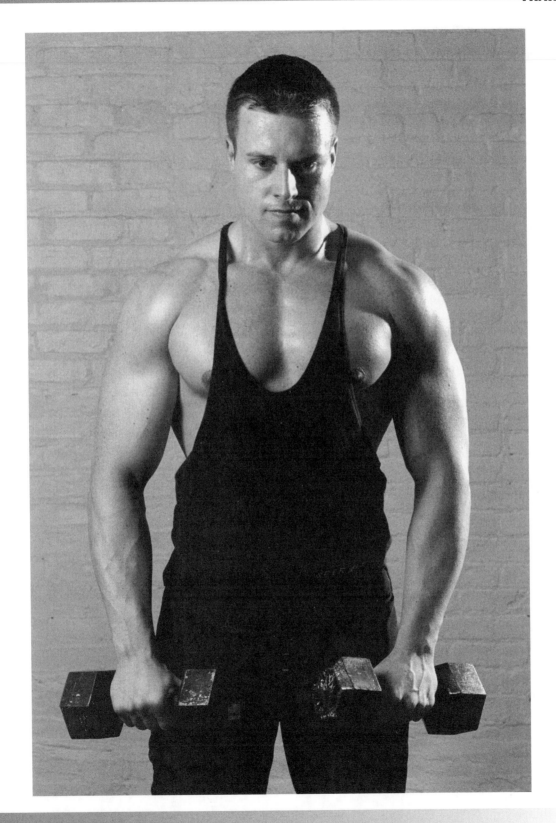

HOW DOES THE 14-DAY BODY SCULPTING WORKOUT WORK?

The 14-Day Body Sculpting Workout is based on your body's physiology. It usually takes your body 14 days to get used to a new practice, whether that practice is a diet, a new exercise program or just getting up earlier in the morning. Getting used to a new practice, such as waking up early to exercise, is a great thing. However, getting used to an exercise program is not as great. Why? Once your body gets used to it, it will stop responding and your results (i.e. fat loss and increased muscle tone) will come to a screeching halt. That is the reason why most people who go to the gym experience great results initially, but later see and feel themselves going nowhere. The key to experiencing continued results is variation. However, it cannot be haphazard variation. You must have a planned scheme that will guarantee continual results; a scheme such as the one offered by the 14-Day Body Sculpting Workout.

For the first two weeks you will use modified compound supersets. During this period, the body gets stronger as rest periods are abundant and repetitions are at a higher range (12-15). Working out this way allows the nervous system to recover and the body to increase its strength. In addition, the high repetitions allow the body to start building more capillaries (necessary for the delivery of nutrients to the muscle cell) and preparing the joints for the heavier weights to come.

On weeks three and four you will start using supersets, a more intense technique that creates higher demands on the central nervous system, along with heavier weights and fewer reps (10-12) with a slightly higher number of sets. The increased volume and the shock to the body created by the increased stress of the weight training routine causes an increased output of growth hormone (a hormone that greatly enhances fat loss and muscle tone), and an increase in metabolism.

When your body starts adapting to this routine, you further increase the intensity by increasing the number of sets again, using heavier weights (8-10 reps) and by using Giant Sets. Once again the body is shocked, growth hormone output goes through the roof and the metabolism is jolted one more time.

The routine is so intense that if you were to maintain it for more than two weeks you would enter a state of overtraining (where your body cannot recover from the demands imposed by the intense routine). When your body has reached a level that gets fairly close to overtraining, you will give your body a chance to recover for the next couple of weeks by going back to week one where you use fewer sets, higher reps and have ample amounts of time to recover in between sets by using the modified compound superset technique. Are you going backwards? Not at all! With this program you are always moving forward. Even though you are going back to a less stressful type of training with less volume, you will notice that you will now be stronger on the same exercises. You will be able to use greater weight for the 12-15 repetition range for the following reason: In order for the body to prevent itself from going into overtraining during the two weeks of high volume and giant sets, it naturally built up its nervous system energies to the highest level possible as an emergency measure. Now that you have backed off on the stress, you'll have all of this extra energy that the body will utilize to get even stronger and more muscular. That is how your strength will increase. Then after two weeks of modified compound supersets, once again you'll begin to increase the stress on the body by continuing this results-producing cycle.

Why is it necessary to get strong and why should you lift heavier weights? Because building up your strength through progressive resistance training is the key to increased muscle tone and accelerated fat loss. Remember, if your strength stays the same, then your body will look the same and you might as well consider yourself moving backwards.

CHOOSING THE BEST TIME TO WORK OUT

We recommend you work out in the morning as soon as you wake up. Drink 16 ounces of cold water before you start the workout and an additional 30 to 60 ounces during the activity. This is essential to prevent dehydration. We recommend working out first thing in the morning on an empty stomach because you will burn 300% more body fat this way. In the morning your body doesn't have any carbohydrates to burn. In the absence of carbohydrates, your body goes straight to the fat stores (triglycerides) in order to get the energy necessary to do the work. Another good reason to work out in the morning is the fact that at this time growth hormone levels are at their highest levels (remember that growth hormone is one of the hormones responsible for muscle growth and the one that influences fat loss the most). Working out in the morning will allow you to expedite the fat loss process for dramatic results. However, we do understand that certain obstacles such as work constraints and other situations might not permit everybody to train in the morning. In this case, do your cardio or weight training three hours after any meal (if your last meal was at 3:00 pm, then your exercise session should be at 6:00 pm).

If you follow the *Advanced 14-Day Body Sculpting Workout* you will be doing Cardio and abs first thing in the morning and weight training at some other time during the day. However, if this is impossible due to your schedule, then perform abs before the weight training workout and cardio right after the weight-training workout is completed. (*Note: If you do decide to workout in the morning, please make sure that you properly warm-up and stretch. This will not only ensure that you are wide awake but will also prevent injuries and potential accidents.*)

WORKOUT CLOTHING

When you go to the gym, you should be wearing comfortable clothes that allow your body to move freely without constraints. Therefore, rigid clothes such as jeans are definitely out of the question. You also need to choose clothes based on the climate you live in and environmental conditions. You should wear extra layers of clothing if your environment is cold helping to keep your body temperature on the warm side and prevent possible injuries. Also wear nice comfortable cross training shoes along with a thick absorbent pair of socks. Never train in your bare feet or with sandals; you could seriously injure your feet if you ever dropped a plate on them.

HOW FAST SHOULD YOU LIFT THE WEIGHT?

Many people in the fitness industry have had difficulty in deciding; "Should I lift the weight fast? Should I lift the weight slow? Should I move the weight fast or slow on the positive (concentric) portion of the rep? Should I move fast or slow on the negative (eccentric) portion of the rep?" We have done the research on these questions and will now explain each one in detail.

We have found that slow lifting is usually only good for beginners who have never lifted a weight. It helps them to learn and master the movement and prevents them from using bad exercise form. However, as you become more advanced, science and our own experience indicate that you should lift the weight as quickly as possible without sacrificing form and without involving momentum (jerking and bouncing of the weights.) You create more force by lifting fast and therefore more muscle fibers need to be activated. By ensuring that you are not using momentum to help you move the weight, you can be sure that the force generated during the movement will be created solely by your muscles and not inertia. This is what helps stimulate your muscles to grow creating the tone and shape that you desire. While some might believe that super slow lifting is beneficial because it is difficult to perform and painful, it is not the best way to stimulate muscle growth. Super slow lifting accumulates too much lactic acid within your muscles and fatigues them before they reach real momentary muscular failure.

Science tells us that Force = Mass (in this case the weight you are lifting) multiplied by Acceleration (the increasing speed at which you lift the weight). Therefore, the best way to lift weights is to lift them fast, with total control of the weight and without relying on momentum. Since you won't be jerking the weights or using ballistic movements during exercise, the risk of getting injured is not any greater than the risk of getting injured lifting slowly.

If you are lifting a weight that only allows you to do 8 repetitions, if you're looking in the mirror, it will look like you are lifting the weight slowly even though you are lifting it as fast as possible. The heavier the weight the slower you will be able to move it, even though you are trying to accelerate it as fast as you can. This is amazing! We are sure you've heard people's concerns about how lifting heavier weights is dangerous, right? It is actually the opposite. When you lift lighter weights, you have the ability to move the weights very

quickly and sloppily because little stress is put upon the muscles, tissues and joints. This creates a greater risk for injuries to occur. When you lift heavier weights, you are forced to go slower with the weights and to use controlled form during movement. Lifting heavier weights will stimulate more muscle fibers while limiting the chance for injuries to occur (assuming that the maximum amount of weight lifted is one that allows for a minimum of 8 repetitions; heavier weights may indeed cause connective tissue injury).

MUSCLE SORENESS

Muscle soreness is caused by micro-trauma to the muscles and is a good indicator that the workout you performed was effective. If you have never exercised before, you will experience higher levels of soreness than usual at the beginning of your program. That is okay. As your body gets used to the exercise program the muscle soreness will subside to tolerable levels. You just need to persevere through those first few weeks. Do not confuse this type of soreness with overtraining.

There are several degrees of soreness that you should be aware of:

- Delayed Onset Muscle Soreness (DOMS)
- Typical Mild Muscle Soreness
- Injury-Type Muscle Soreness

The first type of soreness is delayed onset muscle soreness (DOMS). The term DOMS refers to the deep muscular soreness usually experienced two days after (not the day after) the exercise has been done. DOMS prevents the total muscular contraction from occurring within a muscle. This type of severe soreness is caused when you either embark on an exercise program for the first time or when you train a body part harder than usual. It can last for a couple of days for an advanced well-conditioned athlete or for as long as a week for a beginner. If this type of soreness is affecting you and it is time to work out again, the best thing to do is not to rest but to exercise the affected body part in an active recovery routine.

In active recovery routines all of the loads are reduced by 50 percent, and the sets are not taken to muscular failure. For example, if you are to perform an exercise for 10 repetitions, divide the weight that you usually use for that exercise by two and that is the weight that you will use for your active recovery routine. Also, stop performing the exercise even though you may not reach muscular failure at the tenth rep. The reason for this type of workout is to restore full movement in the muscle, helping to remove the lactic acid and other waste products building up within the muscles. It also forces high concentrations of blood into the damaged area of the muscles and nourishes the muscles for repair and growth. We find that doing this is always beneficial; by the next day you will not be as sore or stiff as you ordinarily would have been if you had skipped a workout in order to wait for the pain to subside.

The second type of soreness is the typical mild muscle soreness experienced the day after a good workout. While scientists are still unable to pinpoint the true cause of such soreness, the explanation generally accepted is that it is caused by micro-trauma at the muscle fiber level and by an excess of lactic acid. At any rate, what's important is that this is good soreness considering it is of a mild nature and muscle function is not impaired as it is with DOMS. The pain generally lasts a day for advanced athletes and up to 3 days for a beginner. This soreness, on average, indicates that you had a good workout the day before because you created the trauma necessary to

trigger adaptation (e.g. muscle growth). When you are no longer experiencing this type of soreness, it is a good indication that your body has successfully adapted to the training program. This is not one of the goals you will be striving for, as it leads to no gains. This is the reason why our program changes on a consistent basis.

The third type of soreness is the one caused by injury. This soreness is entirely different in nature from the ones described above, as it is usually immobilizing and triggers very sharp pain within the muscles and/or joints. Depending on the nature of the injury, the pain might either be experienced constantly or only when the joints are moved or the muscles contract. These injuries often become apparent as soon as they happen. Other times they appear either the day after and even sometimes days after the activity. If you suddenly become injured, the first thing that you should do is apply the RICE principle (Rest, Ice, Compression and Elevation).

After consulting a doctor, they might allow you to continue training, carefully working around the injury (in other words, utilizing exercises that work around the injured muscle(s), without over stepping the range of motion that triggers the pain). More serious injuries, such as a muscle tear, may involve complete rest of the injured and surrounding areas and, depending on the severity, possibly surgery. The best way to prevent this type of injury, pain and soreness, is by cycling your exercise parameters and by constantly practicing good form.

BREATHING WHILE PERFORMING AN EXERCISE

The correct way to breathe while performing an exercise is to exhale while you are forcing the weight up (the concentric phase or muscle contraction) and to inhale while you are lowering or releasing the weight (the eccentric phase or the negative portion of the exercise). For example, if you are doing a bench press, you exhale while you push the weight up away from your body and inhale while you lower the weight down towards your chest.

WARMING UP BEFORE TRAINING AND STRETCHING

People always ask us, "What is the best time for stretching?" Our answer is, the best time for stretching would be after your body temperature has increased and the blood has begun circulating within the muscle. This is achieved by performing exercise that raises your heart rate and circulates the blood at an increased rate. If you fail to adequately do this, you run the risk of tearing a muscle or causing bodily injury. Are you up for an experiment? Wet a rubber band with water and put it in the freezer. After two hours, take it out and try to stretch it to its limit. Pay attention and you will discover that the rubber band easily breaks. The same process can easily happen to your muscles if you stretch them without sufficiently warming them up. Having said that, before you begin the weight training workout, spend 15 minutes warming up followed by light stretching. Just go through the next few steps.

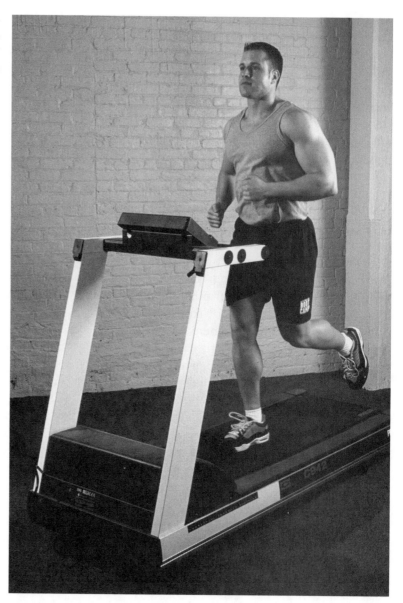

Perform approximately six minutes worth of **aerobic activity** to get the blood flowing and to increase your body temperature.

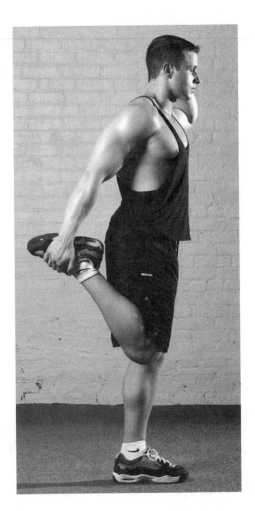

Stretch your **thighs** by grasping a pole with one arm and bending the opposite leg, bringing your foot toward your buttocks (if you grasp the pole with the left hand, then bend the right leg). Grasp your ankle with the free hand and slowly lift your foot as comfortably as possible. Hold this position for a count of 5 and repeat with the other leg.

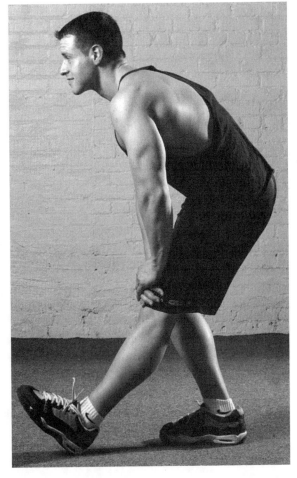

Stretch your **hamstrings** by stepping forward with your left heel while bending your right knee. Keep your left leg straight and toe pointed up. Placing your hands on your left thigh, bend forward at the waist and feel the stretch in your hamstring. Hold this position for a count of five and repeat with the opposite leg.

Stretch your **chest** by grasping a stationary pole with one of your arms, ensuring that this arm is parallel to the ground. Slowly turn away from the pole and allow your arm to be as far behind the body as possible. Ensure that you do not overextend your chest by just going as far away as is comfortably possible. Hold this position for a count of 5 and repeat with the other arm.

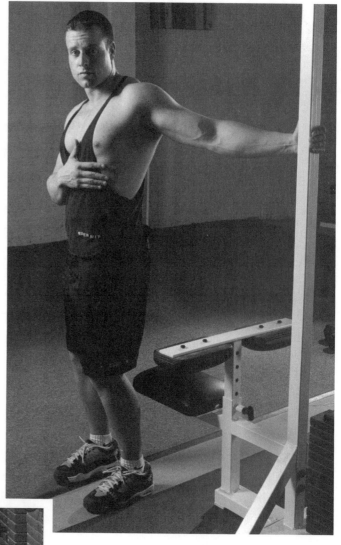

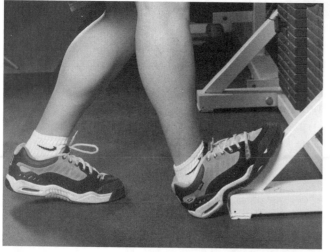

Stretch your **calves** by grasping a pole with both arms, standing on a raised surface, and placing one foot on the edge of the surface in order to allow your heel to go down as far as comfortably possible. Hold this position for a count of 5 and repeat with the other leg.

Stretch your **back** by grasping a pole with both arms, bending your knees, and sitting back in order to fully extend your arms and achieve a stretch in your lats and lower back. Hold this position for a count of 5.

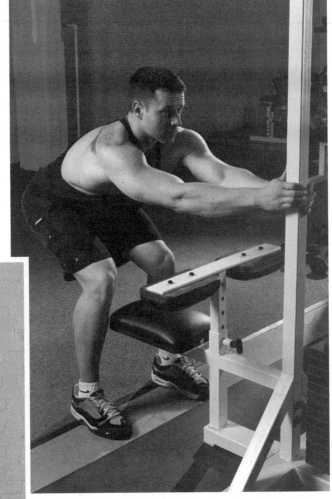

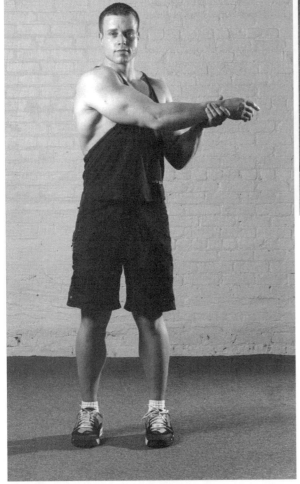

Stretch your **shoulders** by grasping one of your wrists with the opposite hand. Without moving your torso, begin to pull your arm as far as possible. Hold this position for a count of 5 and repeat with the other arm.

SELECTING THE WEIGHT FOR EACH EXERCISE

The weight you select for each exercise depends on the amount of repetitions that you need to do for a particular set. If you need to do between 10-12 repetitions for one set, then you need to pick a weight where you fail (the point at which completing another repetition becomes impossible) between 10-12 reps. This takes a bit of practice but after a while you will become extremely accurate when it comes to choosing the correct weight for a particular repetition range. If you pick a weight that allows you to do more than 12 repetitions, you'll need to increase the amount of weight being lifted. If you reach failure before hitting the tenth rep, you'll need to decrease the amount of weight being lifted. For example, if you were doing 4 sets of an exercise, as you continue to work through the sets, fatigue will set in and you may not be able to continue using the weight that you chose to lift during the first set. When you get to the point where you can no longer lift a particular weight for a pre-determined repetition range, simply decrease the weight and prepare yourself for the next set.

OVERTRAINING

Overtraining is a condition caused when the body is taxed beyond its ability to recover. The main causes may include long workouts, an overload of training volume (too many sets and reps), a bad diet lacking nutrients, lack of sleep, etc. People experiencing this condition might notice such symptoms as a loss of muscle mass, weakness, trouble sleeping, loss of appetite, a lethargic and constant tired feeling, and feelings of depression.

It is impossible to overtrain with our weight training program (assuming you follow the nutrition and rest practices prescribed) because after you stress the body's recuperative capabilities to the maximum (by doing supersets for two weeks and then moving on to Giant Sets for two more), you back off into the less stressful modified compound supersets. In addition, you get a rest day after every day of lifting (unless you are using the advanced version) and you also get the weekends off. During rest days, you concentrate on fat burning aerobic exercise (which aids in the recuperation process by removing the lactic acid created by weight training) instead. We use Sunday as our total inactivity day; you can choose any day of the week as your rest day. This day serves to rest the body and the mind. Finally, the ample nutrients provided by the diet, along with the recommended supplements, eliminate the possibility of getting overtrained.

Provided that you follow the training program as laid out, in conjunction with the nutrition and rest components, overtraining is a state of mind and does not exist.

SKIPPING WORKOUTS

Skipping workouts is unacceptable. You hear it all the time, people constantly making excuses about how they have no time to exercise. Unless you are in a situation where you are on call 24 hours a day and are being utilized at least 23 hours out of the 24, then we are more than sure that you can find the time to train. The fact of the matter is that some people don't want to spend the time exercising, so instead, they make excuses about how busy they are. We don't care if you only have 15 minutes to allocate towards exercise, it's still 15 minutes of exercise! If you are interested in completely changing the way you look and feel, all the excuses in the world can not hold you back from doing what it takes to fit a workout into your schedule. All you need is the vision, the motivation and the determination to do so.

Skipping workouts will severely jeopardize your toning and fat burning efforts, in addition to destroying your bodysculpter's mindset. However, if for some reason you are not able to train (let's say because all the gyms in the world are closed on that day, and you have no gym at home and don't know anyone with one), then remember back to what your grandparents used to say, about how they had to walk over 5 miles just to get to work, in the snow, with no shoes or socks! In all seriousness, if you skip a workout one day, simply make up the skipped session the next day. This might mean training twice in one day (doing your cardio session in the morning and weights in the afternoon) or sacrificing your Sunday rest day. If you skip a workout for whatever reason, don't beat yourself up about it. Just realize that tomorrow is a new day and you will be able to make up the skipped session. However, don't make a habit of skipping training sessions, as skipping sessions will ultimately limit the results you expect to receive.

Chapter 4
Nutrition

4

THE **BODY**
SCULPTING
BIBLE
FOR **MEN**

The second component of the formula for body-sculpting success is nutrition. Nutrition provides the raw materials for energy, growth and recuperation. Without a sufficient diet, it will be impossible to achieve your goal of building an ideal body.

If you truly wish to fulfill all of your body-sculpting goals—quickly—you must follow the nutritional guidelines that we will discuss. Too many people neglect these guidelines and consequently, they fail to create a beautiful physique. You can train as though you were a super hero and get all of the necessary sleep and rest, but if you don't eat correctly, you will falter. If, on the other hand, you train to the best of your ability, receive adequate sleep and rest, and eat the right foods, **watch out!** The right balance of these three components will give you your ideal body in no time.

Any discussion of a good nutrition program begins with the nutrition basics.

NUTRITION BASICS

To function properly, the body needs the following three macronutrients:

CARBOHYDRATES

Carbohydrates are your body's main source of energy. When you ingest carbohydrates, your pancreas releases a hormone called insulin. Insulin is very important because:

- It attaches to the carbohydrates and stores them in the muscles or stores them as fat.

- It grabs on to the amino acids (the building blocks of proteins) and stores them in the muscle cell so that they can be used for recovery and repair.

Ironically, most overweight people are on low-fat/high-carbohydrate diets are in that condition because they consume too many carbs. An overabundance of carbohydrates causes your body to release excessive amounts of insulin. When too much insulin is present, your body converts the extra carbohydrate calories into fat, creating a human fat-storing machine. It is therefore imperative that we eat the optimal amount of carbs—not too many and not too few.

Having established the importance of carbohydrates in your diet, let's discuss which foods are the best sources of carbs.

Carbohydrates are divided into two categories: complex carbs and simple carbs. The complex carbs provide sustained or "timed released" energy, while the simple carbs give you immediate energy. We recommend that you eat mainly complex carbs throughout the day, because they provide consistent energy levels for peak performance and daily functions. Simple carbs, for which fruits are a primary source, are best consumed 20 to 30 minutes after a workout, when your body needs to replenish its glycogen levels immediately. This will help reduce the recuperation time and aid in the production of lean muscle tissue. Ingesting simple carbs throughout the day is not recommended because they are released into the bloodstream too quickly, and if you do not need them at that specific time, your body's insulin will help to store them as body fat.

We are not limiting fruits because they are unhealthy; they are indeed very healthy and provide several essential vitamins and minerals. We limit them because they tend to slow fat loss. Fructose, the sugar contained in fruits, is easily stored as body fat, and the carbs from most fruits are released into the bloodstream too quickly causing a sharp rise in insulin.

Some simple carbs are released into the bloodstream more quickly than others. Those with a high glycemic index are the fastest and should be eaten only immediately after workouts.

There are two types of complex carbohydrates: starchy and fibrous. Following are lists of the best sources for each, as a well as lists of the best sources for higher and lower glycemic index simple carbs:

COMPLEX CARBOHYDRATES

(Eat in small portions throughout the day)

- Starchy: oatmeal, potatoes, grits, brown rice, lentils, sweet potatoes, whole-wheat bread, chickpeas and pitas.

- Fibrous: asparagus, squash, broccoli, green beans, cabbage, cauliflower, celery, cucumbers, mushrooms, lettuce, red or green peppers, tomatoes, spinach, and zucchini.

SIMPLE CARBOHYDRATES

(Eat sparingly, primarily after exercising, especially the high-glycemic index carbs. Limit yourself to two servings a day.)

- High-Glycemic Index: bananas, grapes and skim milk (which also contains protein

- Lower-Glycemic Index: apples, pears, cantaloupes, oranges, cherries, strawberries, grapefruits, lemons, nectarines and peaches.

PROTEIN

Every tissue in your body (muscle, hair, skin, nails, etc.) consists of protein.

Proteins are also the building blocks of lean muscle tissue. Their role is paramount. Without protein, building muscle and burning fat efficiently would be impossible. Protein helps increase your metabolism by 20 percent every time you eat food containing it, and it time-releases carbohydrates in the form of glucose so that you have energy throughout the day.

While following the 14-Day Body Sculpting Program, you should consume from 1 to 1.5 grams of protein per pound of lean body mass. In other words, if you are 130 pounds with 16 percent body fat, you should consume at least 109 grams of protein, because your lean body mass equals 109 pounds. Most people should not consume more than 1.5 grams per pound of lean body mass because any extra protein that is not converted into glucose and used for energy or excreted will provide excess calories. While it is very unlikely that protein itself will be stored as fat, a consistent caloric intake greater than that required by your body will eventually lead to an increase in fat.

PROTEIN SOURCES

Following is a list of some of the best sources for protein: salmon, halibut, cod, round steak, chicken breast, tuna (packed in water), sardines, turkey breast, whey protein, egg substitutes, and skim milk (which also contains simple carbs and ideally should be limited to post workout consumption).

FATS

All of the cells in the body contain some fat. Fats are responsible for lubricating your joints. In addition, hormones are manufactured from fats. If you eliminate all fats from your diet, your hormonal production will drop, and an array of chemical reactions will be interrupted. Because your testosterone production is halted, the production of lean muscle mass will also cease. Your body will start accumulating more body fat than usual to keep functioning.. Therefore, to maintain an efficient metabolism, we need to consume certain fats.

There are three types of fats: Saturated, which are associated with high cholesterol and heart disease; polyunsaturated, which don't affect cholesterol levels; and monounsaturated, which raise good cholesterol levels.

Following are the best (and worse) sources for the various types of fats

Saturated fats: These are associated with high cholesterol levels and heart disease and are commonly found in animal products such as. However, some vegetable fats are altered in a chemical process known as hydrogenation that increases their levels of saturated fats. Hydrogenated vegetable oils are generally found in packaged foods. In addition, coconut oil, palm oil, and palm kernel oil—which are also frequently used in packaged foods—and non-dairy creamers contain high levels of saturated fats.

Polyunsaturated fats: These fats do not affect cholesterol levels. The fats in corn oil, cottonseed oil, safflower oil, soybean oil, and sunflower oil are polyunsaturated.

Monounsaturated fats: These fats raise your levels of the good cholesterol. They are usually high in essential fatty acids and may contain beneficial antioxidant properties. Sources of these fats include fish oils, virgin olive oil, canola oil, flaxseed oil, safflower oil and nat-ural peanut butter. We refer to these types of fats as good fats.

Good fats should comprise 20 percent of your caloric intake. Less than 20 percent will reduce your hormonal production. More than 20 percent will lead to an accumulation of fat.

WATER

Water is by far the most abundant substance in our body. Without water, an organism would not survive. Most people who come to us for advice on how to get in shape underestimate the value of water.

Water is essential for the following reasons:

- More than 65 percent of your body is composed of water, including most of your muscle cells.

- As it is excreted, water removes from your body.

- Water is necessary for all of the complex chemical reactions that your body performs on a daily basis. Processes such as energy production, muscle building, and fat burning all require water. A lack of water interrupts all of these functions.

- Water helps lubricate the joints, increasing mobility and decreasing joint pain.

- When external temperatures rise, water serves as a coolant that maintains the body temperature at the appropriate level.

- Water helps control your appetite. Have you ever felt hungry after eating a huge meal? This might be an indication that your body is beginning to dehydrate. If you drink water at this time, your cravings will stop.

- Cold water increases your metabolism and aids in the breakdown of body fat.

HOW MUCH SHOULD I DRINK?

To determine how much water your body needs each day, multiply your lean body mass by 0.66. This figure will represent how many ounces of water your body requires on a daily basis to function optimally.

CHARACTERISTICS OF A GOOD NUTRITION PROGRAM

To create a diet that will help you meet your body-sculpting goals, you will need to follow these nutritional guidelines.

Your nutrition plan should be based on eating small and frequent meals throughout the day. Such a plan will greatly increase the speed of your metabolism. Consider how your car uses gasoline as an energy source to maintain its performance. It consumes only as much fuel as it needs, and the farther you drive, the more gas your car needs. Your body functions in a similar fashion, using food as its energy source while efficiently burning fat. While it is commonly perceived that an extreme reduction in calories is the key to losing fat, the truth is that if you go more than three or four hours without eating, your body switches to a catabolic state, a condition in which you lose muscle and gain fat. Your body believes that it is starving and reacts by cannibalizing lean muscle tissue. It also feeds on your body's water supply and organ tissue

while storing calories as fat for future use. Needless to say, this is a bad scenario.

Other reasons for eating frequent meals involve blood sugar, insulin management, and energy levels. Large infrequent feedings result in greater releases of insulin, which in turn lead to blood-sugar crashes and low energy levels 30 minutes to an hour after the meal. In addition, whatever calories the body cannot use at that time are stored as body fat for future use. Also, the lethargy that accompanies low blood-sugar levels can create cravings for sweets. Small frequent feedings spike the metabolism and maintain a consistent blood-sugar level that results in better utilization of nutrients, more stable energy, and fewer or no cravings throughout the day.

With the 14-Day Body Sculpting Program, you will be eating five or six meals a day (six or seven if you are following The Advanced 14-Day Body Sculpting Program) at 2-1/2- to three-hour intervals.

Your meals should include the optimal ratios of carbohydrates to protein to fat. Avoid meals that don't have the proper balance of nutrients, such as an all-carbohydrate meal of pasta. Every macronutrient has to be present for the body to absorb and use efficiently. Without delving too deeply into biochemistry, rest assured that if you eat a meal that consists only of carbohydrates, your energy level will crash in about 30 minutes, and your body will store as fat any carbs that were not used. Conversely, if you eat only protein, you will lack the energy supplied by carbs, and your body will not be able to convert the protein into lean muscle tissue. Your body has difficultly absorbing protein in the absence of carbs, because scarce amounts of insulin are available to carry the amino acids from the protein into the muscle cell. In addition, the ratios for each particular macronutrient have to be correct to produce the results that you desire.

Do not smoke and limit your alcohol consumption. Tobacco and alcohol reduce testosterone levels, in addition to causing many other health problems. Alcohol in particular can be responsible for gaining fat because each gram of alcohol contains seven calories.

Increase your intake of protein. Proteins are the building blocks of all living organisms. Just as you would need more raw material to construct a skyscraper than to build a house, you require additional protein for body sculpting. Several researchers have concluded that the protein needs of people engaged in weight training exceed those of sedentary people. While researchers continue to debate just how much more, most of us in the personal training field agree that 1 to 1.5 grams of protein per lean body mass is optimal for anyone engaged in intense training. "What about kidney damage?" some may ask. Concerns that high levels of protein adversely affect the kidney was refuted by a study, "Do Regular High Protein Diets Have Potential Health Risks on Kidney Function in Athletes?" which was published in 2000 in the *International Journal of Sports Nutrition.* The study's authors, Jacques R. Poortmans and Oliver Dellalieux, concluded that higher protein intakes do not pose a threat to healthy kidney function. However, their findings do not apply to people suffering from a pre-existing kidney condition.

Reduce your intake of bad fats and bring on the good fats. Bad fats, or saturated fats, are found in butter, cooking oils, and red meats. Good fats, or monounsaturated fats, are those contained in such foods as flaxseed oil, extra virgin olive oil, and natural peanut butter. One tablespoon a day of flaxseed oil fulfills most people's essential fatty acid requirements. I tend to take one tablespoon in the morning with my protein shake. You can also divide your intake of good fats into three teaspoons taken over the course of the day.

Reduce your intake of sugars. Foods laden

COOKING TIPS

Proper food preparation is essential for achieving your body-sculpting goals

- Eat vegetables raw or slightly steamed. If boiling vegetables, be careful not to overcook or them. If you do, you will lose all of the nutritients.

- Never fry. Broil, grill, steam or bake. Broiling, grilling and steaming are the preferred cooking methods because they allow fat to drain while cooking.

- Trim all fat from meat and remove skin from poultry prior to cooking.

- Do not use salts, butter, oils, or sugar when cooking. Instead, experiment with herbs, non-salt seasonings, lemon juice, vinegar, garlic and pepper, even a touch (1 tablespoon) of white or red wine. The occasional use of salsa, low-sodium soy sauce, catsup, or mustard to enhance the flavor of meats and vegetables is okay if they are used sparingly (1 tablespoon at the most). Minced white or green onions are also excellent for seasoning.

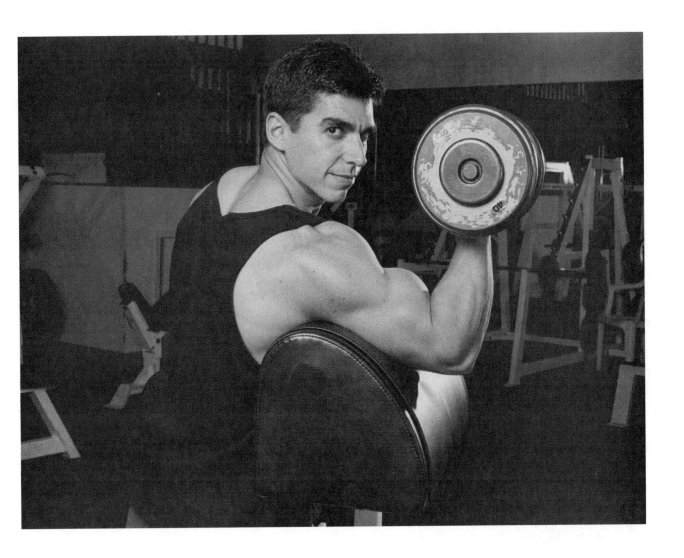

with sugar cause a sharp rise in insulin levels. Insulin is a beneficial hormone when it is not present in excessive amounts because it carries the amino acids from the protein into the muscle cells, where it is used for growth and repair. It also carries carbohydrates into the liver and muscle cells, where they can be stored as glycogen and used in the future. However, once the body's carbohydrate storage capacity is full, insulin turns these carbs into fat.

In addition, excessive insulin production will remove the carbs from the blood stream too quickly, creating a low blood-sugar level that leaves you feeling groggy and usually craving sweets. It is a vicious cycle that ultimately leads to fat gain. The best way to avoid this cycle is to eliminate all junk food from your diet, ridding your body of empty calories that are not used and eventually turned into fat. Foods that are high in sugars and fats are the worst for your body because when both of these macronutrients are present it is

extremely easy for insulin to carry these triglycerides (fats) into the adipose tissue stores (fat cells). Non-diet sodas as well as fruit juices should also be eliminated from your diet. Like sodas, most fruit juices have very high sugar contents, typically 30 to 40 grams per 8-ounce serving. Four servings a day will supply most of your daily carbohydrate needs in the form of bad calories, ones that will not be used as efficiently as those from complex, slow-releasing sources such as oatmeal.

Eat the right foods after a workout. The most important meal is the post-workout meal. It should consist of simple carbs or high glycemic complex carbs and preferably a fast-release liquid protein such as whey isolate. Include a minimum of fat and fiber in the meal because both reduce the speed at which the food is absorbed. A good post-workout meal could include skim milk with a banana and whey isolate protein powder. Whey isolate protein is especially suitable because it is released

BEVERAGE TIPS

Because they lack knowledge of nutrition, many dieters can ruin their diets without realizing it. Beverages are often the culprits. Here is some advice that will help you avoid or overcome bad drinking habits.

- Drink plenty of water daily. For each pound of your weight, you should drink 2/3 of an ounce daily. In other words, if you weight 200 pounds, we recommend that you drink 132 ounces of water a day.

- Eliminate all non-diet sodas and fruit juices, even those that claim to be all-natural. These beverages contain too many simple carbs. For example, the average 12-ounce soda contains 40 grams of sugar, while an 8-ounce serving of the average fruit juice contains from 25 to 35 grams of simple carbs.

- Crystal Lite beverages and decaffeinated tea or coffee are okay as long as they are consumed in moderation; your primary beverage should be water.

- Avoid alcohol, though an occasional glass of red wine is okay, provided that you are of legal drinking age.

into the bloodstream very quickly, and it contains no fats that would slow the digestive process. Cream of is another good carbohydrate to consume after a workout. While it is not a simple carbohydrate, it does have a high glycemic index, meaning that it will create the high levels of insulin needed for glycogen replenishment after a workout. An ideal post-workout meal could consist of 1/3 cup of uncooked cream of rice mixed with whey protein isolate. This combination will replenish all glycogen stores immediately and provide the body with the amino acids that it needs.

CALORIC AND MACRONUTRIENT INTAKE

In this section we will discuss how much of the nutrients from each category you should consume, beginning with a description of the formula for calculating your lean body mass.

Lean Body Mass, or LBM equals your total weight minus your fat weight. You can calculate your fat weight by using a pair of skin fold calipers or by having a trainer at your health club (if you are a member) check it for you. You can also refer to **Appendix F**: Tracking your Progress, where we present some formulas that you can use.

The optimal diet consists of 40 percent carbs, 40 percent protein, and 20 percent fats.

CALORIC REQUIREMENTS

Caloric requirements for most men fluctuate from roughly 2000 to 2500 calories per day. However, if you eat the same amount of calories every day, your body will become accustomed to that amount, and you will stop losing fat. Therefore, we recommend that you alternate between 2000 and 2500 calories; for two weeks, consume 2000 calories, and then the following two weeks consume 2500. We will

discuss this concept further in the **<tk>** section.

Once you know the total amount of calories you need to take in every day, calculate the amount (in grams) of each nutrient by using the aforementioned percentages. Here is how to do that:

Total amount of carbs for the day = (Total number of calories x 0.40)/ 4

Total amount of protein for the day = (Total number of calories x 0.40)/ 4

Total amount of fat for the day = (Total number of calories x 0.20)/ 9

We divide the carbs and proteins by 4 because each gram of carbs and protein contains 4 calories. For fats, we divide by 9 because there are 9 calories in every gram of fat.

Dividing each of the sums from these formulas by a factor of 5 (by a factor of 6 if you are eating six meals a day) gives you the amount of each nutrient that you will need to consume per meal. While it isn't necessary to include the exact amount of each nutrient with every meal, you do want to make sure that you stay within 10 grams (plus or minus) of the formula when counting protein and carbs and within 5 grams (plus or minus) when counting fats.

Appendix C offers a diet plan in which all of these calculations have been completed. To alter the menu, simply substitute comparable choices for the foods listed.

CHOOSING WHAT TO EAT

Now that you have calculated the amount of carbs, protein and fats you need for each meal, you still have to choose what foods to eat. This is one of the greatest challenges that we face when beginning a diet, but the food-group tables on the following pages can assist with these decisions. They include the nutritional levels for each of the foods that we recommend.

Although the tables are accurate, they do not address all of the alterations that can occur during food processing. If you discover a discrepancy between the nutritional information on a food label and that which is included in the chart, defer to the food label.

WHAT IF I DON'T WANT TO DO THE CALCULATIONS?

No problem. In **Appendix C**, we have included diet charts in which the figures have already been calculated. This appendix provides two sample diets (one with 2000 calories and another one with 2500 calories) that have taken into consideration all of the guidelines presented above. If you want to alternate a food item, go to **Appendix B**, which contains a copy of the food tables on page 73. You can use these tables to find a substitute that contains a similar amount of nutrients.

WHAT IF I DON'T WANT TO GO ON A DIET?

Whether you eat candy or carrots all day everyday, this is your nutritional diet. Usually people associate diets with starvation and days of agony. However, this is not the correct characterization of the term. The word diet refers to the food choices that we make on a daily basis. In this book, we are going to present you with a program that you will be able to use for the rest of your life to remain in tip-top shape. Our diet works because of the food choices, the frequency of meals, and the intentional fluctuations in caloric intake. We don't expect you to change overnight. In fact, most dieters fail because they attempt to make immediate dras-

tic changes. Most of those who succeed do so by making incremental progressive changes that eventually bring them to their goals. This is how we are going to teach you to change your diet, with small incremental steps that will yield huge rewards.

BABY STEPS, GIANT RESULTS: THE NO-PAIN, ALL-GAIN PLAN TO A PERFECT DIET

In keeping with our 14-day philosophy, we will make incremental changes to your diet every two weeks. Remember that this is how long it takes to create a new pattern as well as how long it takes the body to get used to something new. Every 14 days we are going to set a new goal, and each of these goals will build upon the success of the previous one. By achieving a new goal every two weeks, you will end up with a diet that will yield the consistent fat loss/muscle toning results you are seeking. In other words, you will have the type of diet that we discussed in the previous section.

WEEKS 1-2: CUT THE FAT.

During the first two weeks, we want you to begin looking at food labels. Start eliminating as many fats as possible from your diet by making some instant changes in your current routine. For example:

- If you fry food, start steaming or broiling it instead.

- If you use salad dressings with high-fat contents, replace them with low-fat or non-fat choices.

- Select meats with less fat. For instance, if you enjoy corned beef, try skinless chicken or turkey instead. If you eat chicken with the skin on,

FOOD GROUP TABLES

For the post-workout meal, choose one item from Group A and 1 item from Group C in order to create a balanced meal. For all other meals, choose one item from Group A, one item from Group B, and 1 item from Group D in order to create a balanced meal. Remember to adjust the serving size depending upon the amount of nutrients that you require per meal (remember your calculations? Go back and figure them out if you haven't already).

GROUP A - PROTEIN			
FOOD	GRAMS	FOOD	GRAMS
Chicken breast (3.5 oz. broiled)	33	White fish (3.5 oz broiled)	31
Tuna (packed in water, 3.5 oz)	35	Halibut (3.5 oz broiled)	31
Turkey breast (3.5 oz broiled)	28	Cod (3.5 oz broiled)	31
Whey protein powder (2 scoops)	22	Round steak (3.5 oz broiled)	33
10 egg whites	35	Top sirloin (4 oz)	35

Note: These weights are for uncooked portions

GROUP B - CARBOHYDRATE (COMPLEX, STARCHY)			
FOOD	GRAMS	FOOD	GRAMS
Baked potato (3.5 oz broiled)	21	Lentils (1 cup dry, cooked)	38
Plain oatmeal (1/2 cup dry)	27	Grits (1/2 cup dry)	31
Whole wheat bread (1 slice; limit if reducing body fat)	13	Pita bread (1 piece)	33
Cream of rice (1/2 cup dry, post workout only)	38	Sweet potato (4 oz)	28
Chickpeas (1 cup cooked)	45	Brown rice (2/3 cup cooked)	30

GROUP C - CARBOHYDRATE (SIMPLE)			
FOOD	GRAMS	FOOD	GRAMS
Apple (1)	15	Banana (6 oz, *post workout only*)	27
Cantaloupe (1/2)	25	Grapes (1 cup, *post workout only*)	14
Strawberries (1 cup)	9	Grapefruit (1/2)	12
Orange (1)	15	Tangerine (1)	9
Pear (1)	27	Cherries (1 cup)	22
Lemon (1)	5	Nectarine (1)	16
Peach (1)	10	Skim milk (1 cup, *preferably post workout only*)	13

GROUP D - CARBOHYDRATE (COMPLEX, FIBROUS)			
FOOD (10 OZ SERVING)	GRAMS	FOOD (10 OZ SERVING)	GRAMS
Asparagus	5	Yellow squash	12
Broccoli	17	Green beans	23
Cabbage	6	Cauliflower	12
Celery	6	Cucumber	7
Mushrooms	6	Lettuce	7
Red or Green peppers	15	Tomato	5
Spinach	3	Zucchini	13

FAST FOOD RECOMMENDATIONS

Each of the major fast food chains includes some healthy meals on its menu. Here are some offerings that we recommend.

Arby's: Light Chicken Deluxe Sandwich with extra lettuce and tomato (no mayo), Light Turkey Deluxe Sandwich, or roast chicken salad (hold the high-fat dressing)

Bennigan's: Chicken platter, which includes two chicken breasts, and a serving of spicy rice and vegetables

Boston Market: Chicken or turkey sandwich; turkey or chicken breast with a small serving of steamed vegetables, potatoes, corn, rice pilaf or fruit salad

Golden Corral: chicken (remove the skin) with steamed rice and green beans

Hardee's: Chicken fillet sandwich or grilled chicken salad

Kentucky Fried Chicken: A quarter chicken (no skin) and a small serving of mashed potatoes, garden rice, or red beans

Long John Silver's: Flavor-baked chicken or fish and a plain baked potato or a small serving of green beans

McDonald's: McGrilled Chicken Classic or a Chunky Chicken Salad

Subway: A small roast turkey breast sub, a veggie sub or a roast beef sub (with no mayo or extra oils)

Taco Bell: A Light Chicken Burrito, a Light Chicken Taco, a Light Bean Burrito, a Light Soft Taco Supreme, a Light Taco Supreme, a Light Taco, or a Light Soft Taco

Wendy's: A grilled chicken sandwich or a grilled chicken salad

If you find yourself in restaurant not included on this list, don't panic. Just order a chicken plate, and remove the skin. If you follow Eating on the Run rules, no matter where you dine, you won't have a problem finding something suitable on the menu. Bon Appetite!

start removing it; chicken skin is very fatty. If you like red meats, buy only the lean cuts.

By the end of the first two-week period, your taste buds will get used to your new low-fat eating habits.

WEEKS 3-4: ELIMINATE REFINED SUGARS.

Refined sugars are everywhere. Therefore, to accomplish this goal, do the following:

- Stop drinking non-diet sodas; they contain large amounts of refined sugars. You can drink diet sodas, however, they contain Aspartame, and that the consequences of consuming high levels of Aspartame over a long period of time remain undetermined.

- Eliminate the use of table sugars.

- Stop eating sweets.

WEEKS 5-6: BEGIN DRINKING ABUNDANT AMOUNTS OF WATER.

Start drinking much more water than you are used to drinking. Here are some tips for accomplishing this goal:

- Substitute water for all types of drinks, including diet sodas and fruit juices, even those that claim to be all natural.

- Whenever you become thirsty, drink water.

- Drink at least an 8-ounce glass of water with every meal.

- Drink approximately 16 ounces or more of water during your workouts.

WEEKS 7-8: CONTROL YOUR CALORIC INTAKE AND MANAGE YOUR MACRONUTRIENT LEVELS.

During these next two weeks, we will move very close to the ideal diet. The good news is that after these two weeks, dieting will not become any more complicated, and you will continue to see some truly incredible results.

To jump on the fast track toward these gains, do the following:

- Follow a diet similar to the Low Calorie Diet outlined in **Appendix C.**

- Maintain a list of everything that you eat, along with the corresponding macronutrient values to ensure that you don't exceed each meal's allotted macronutrient intake as explained in **Appendix B**.

The Caloric Cycling section that follows offers instructions on how to proceed with your diet after week 8.

CALORIC CYCLING

Congratulations for making it this far. By now, thanks to the training and the diet, you are noticing some extremely favorable changes in the way that you look and feel. The secret for creating even more powerful and consistent results is caloric cycling. By incorporating the following cycling principles into your diet, you'll never stall at the weight-loss plateaus that most dieters encounter.

In the training section **Chapter 3**, we discussed how the body will quickly adapt to an exercise program and stop responding to the routine. When this happens, you stop seeing results; your efforts become wasted. The same principle applies to your diet.

Caloric cycling will play an essential role in keeping your metabolism burning fat efficiently and in toning your body. In fact, recent research indicates that by cycling your calories you can double the rate at which you lose fat.

Here's how to cycle calories:

- Refer to **Appendix C** and follow the High Calorie Diet for two weeks.

- Follow the Low Calorie Diet found in **Appendix C** for the next two weeks.

- Continue to alternate these diets every two weeks.

- Continue to list everything that you eat as well as the foods' macronutrient values to ensure that you don't exceed each meal's allotted macronutrient levels.

STRIVE FOR CONSISTENCY, NOT PERFECTION

We often see dieters who do great at the beginning but eventually they miss a workout or deviate from their diet. They then become discouraged and continue missing workouts or sabotaging their diet. Weeks may pass before they get back on track—if they ever do. Meanwhile, their muscle tone fades, and the fat pounds pile up. Remember, we are all human, and we are entitled to make mistakes. Always strive for perfection, but if for some reason things don't go as well as they should on a given day, forget about it and jump right back into your program the next day. If you eat a bad meal, don't compound the problem by eating incorrectly for the rest of the day. If you miss a workout, don't wait until the following week to resume your routine. The next day, pick up from where you left off. In the end,

your determination and consistency will enable you to win the battle of the bulge.

TROUBLESHOOTING YOUR CALORIC INTAKE

The optimum fat-loss rate is two pounds per week. If you shed more than two pounds, you will lose muscle and muscle tone, yielding a saggy appearance and a significantly slower metabolism. Having said that, we should point out that while most men burn from 2000 to 2500 calories a day, some have a faster-than-normal metabolism. Therefore, some men lose more than two pounds a week at the prescribed number of calories, and others may gain weight. If you find yourself in either situation, don't panic. If you are losing too much, simply add 300 calories to both the lower-calorie diet and the higher-calorie diet, so that your diet alternates between 2300 and 2800 calories. After two weeks, measure your lean body mass to assess how well this plan is working. If you are still losing too much weight after two weeks, increase your calories by an additional 300 for another two weeks. Continue to increase your diet by 300-calorie increments every two weeks until you reach the caloric intake that allows for a 2-pound fat loss while at the same time adding muscle tone.

If you are gaining weight, decrease your calories by 150 for both the lower-calorie diet and the higher-calorie diet. If you find that you are still gaining after the 150-calorie cut, reduce your caloric intake by an additional 150. Don't jump the gun, though. Give your body the two-week opportunity to adjust before decreasing your calories.

EATING ON THE RUN: FAST FOODS

The fast pace of our lives can tax our abilities to plan and prepare for everything, including meals. If time constraints don't allow you to prepare all of the food you need for the day, or if you simply run out of food, there is a solution. You can visit a fast food restaurant. Fast foods are not necessarily bad if you are trying to get in shape, as long as you make wise selections from the menus and follow these rules:

- If this is not your cheat day (see The **Sunday Reward** section), refrain from

choosing fatty foods such as French fries.

- Drink 8 to 16 ounces of water before you arrive at the restaurant and then drink an additional 8 to 16 ounces with your meal. This will prevent you from feeling hungry and succumbing to temptation. If temptation is strong remember that there is nothing better than being in shape, and that you control everything that goes into your

THE RULES IN CHOOSING FOODS

When selecting the components of a meal, you need to follow these guidelines:

- Always try to use natural foods. Avoid using canned or prepared foods because they usually contain too much sodium and too many fats, and carbs.

- Stay within 10 grams (plus of minus) of the recommended amount of carbs and proteins. For fats, stay within 5 grams (plus or minus).

- Always choose low-fat protein sources. If you eat very low-fat meals, don't worry about suffering a fat deficiency, because the supplements program addresses essential fatty acids needs. Bear in mind also that trace amounts of fats are present even in the low-fat protein sources that we recommend.

- If you include skim milk in your diet, remember that it contains protein (8 to 9 grams for every 8 ounces of milk) as well as simple carbs (12 to 13 grams for every 8 ounces of milk). Therefore, count milk as both. Note that because the carbs in milk are simple carbs, you should include it only in post-workout meals. If, because of your schedule, your diet includes protein shakes, and the carbs that you rely on are those found in skim milk, add a teaspoon of flaxseed oil to each shake; the oil will slow the release of the simple carbs into the blood stream. If you plan to participate in body building competitions, eliminate all dairy products from your diet. These foods tend to make you retain water, and the lactose in them makes it difficult to reach the low body-fat percentage required when competing. Your consumption of whole-wheat products should also be minimized while training for competition because they may contain pythoestrogens that would make it more difficult to lose fat.

- Try to include fibrous carbs in at least two meals.

- Post-workout meals should include high-glycemic carbs combined with fast release proteins such as whey protein isolate. Eliminate fats and fibers from this meal.

mouth. Food does not and should not control you.

- Always combine a serving of low-fat protein (in the case of fast food restaurants, this is either skinless chicken or turkey) with a small serving of carbs. Remember that when you eat a chicken or turkey sandwich, the bread counts as the carbs.

- Salads—in addition to a serving of protein and a serving of starchy carbs—are always a good choice because they provide fiber, and they fill you up. However, avoid high-fat or high-sugar dressings.

- Refrain from using high-carbohydrate sauces or mayonnaise.

DO I NEED TO MEASURE MY FOOD INTAKE AND LOG IT IN A DIARY FOREVER?

No, you don't. You will likely notice that after the first eight-week cycle, you know how much food you need to eat everyday. However, without keeping track at the beginning of the program, it would be impossible to determine the correct quantity of nutrients your body needs to lose weight and tone up. Once you establish your food requirements, you can start building your meals based on visual inspections alone, but be careful not to progressively put more food on the plate. If you notice that your weight is climbing, track your food intake for the next three days and determine how far you are deviating from the amounts that you should be eating.

THE SUNDAY REWARD

We want you to cheat on your diet for one meal each Sunday, that is to say, we want you to forget about counting calories and eat whatever you want—within reason, of course. You can reward yourself in this way only if you have stayed on track the rest of the week. One cheat meal a week is actually beneficial because it confuses your body and increases your metabolism. By cheating, you prevent your body from adjusting to the diet, which would lower your metabolism. It also removes the psychological fear that you will never again be able to eat bad foods. Having said that, we must caution that some people (ourselves included) find it difficult to resume a good diet if they eat cheat foods once a week. They binge these foods for weeks at a time. Don't feel bad if you fall into this category. It is natural to crave foods that are bad. After all, they taste so darn good. If you don't think you can limit yourself to just one cheat meal, then stick to a healthy diet and stay away from cheat meals until you feel more confident about your will power.

THE IMPORTANCE OF PREPARING FOOD BEFOREHAND

Preparation is crucial to the success of your dietary program. **If you are not prepared, you will fail.** Life is too hectic to be able to eat four or five times a day without some preparation.

You can prepare your food the night before and store it in containers that have sections for complex or simple carbs, fibrous carbs, and protein. You also can prepare protein shakes ahead of time. The next day, all you have to do is remove the breakfast container from the refrigerator, heat it, and eat. Then grab the container for lunch and two protein shakes, put them in a cooler, and go to work. Also, remember to take a water bottle everywhere you go. There is no need to dehydrate while at work. When you come home, take out the container holding dinner, re-heat the food, eat it, and prepare your meals for the next day.

If you think you will be able to stick to the plan without being prepared, you're taking a risk. You will either end up eating the wrong kinds of food or missing meals. And you will definitely spend more money, because eating out is not cheap.

MEAL FREQUENCY AND WORK

Choose from among these plans to make sure you have five or six meals a day:

- Have complete meals for lunch and dinner and substitute meal-replacement protein shakes or protein bars for the other meals.

- Eat a complete meal for breakfast, lunch and dinner and meal-replacement protein shakes for the other two meals.

- Convince your boss to give you three 20-minute breaks instead of an hour lunch break so that you can eat complete meals throughout the work day and at home.

A WORD ABOUT PROTEIN SHAKES

It's better to eat as much real food as possible. If you are too busy to prepare four to six complete meals a day, try replacing some with protein shakes. You can have a meal-replacement packet mixed with water or a scoop of protein mixed in skim milk with a teaspoon of flaxseed oil. However, be sure to eat at least two complete meals a day.

EMOTIONAL EATING

In our fast-paced, high-stress society, many people resort to emotional eating for comfort. This can be dangerous if it happens too often because the weight will begin to pile on, especially if this eating pattern occurs at night after work.

Remember that you need to list everything you eat during the first eight weeks of this program. During this period, it should be easier to resist the temptation to comfort yourself with food because you will have to document it in your log. If you are past the original eight weeks, then ask yourself, "Am I eating this because my body needs, it or is it because I need it emotionally?" If it's the latter, stop and think about what is most important for you. Is it the food or is it your fitness goals? You know what the right choice is. If it's late at night, just go to bed and rest assured that the cravings will have gone away by morning.

EATING TO GAIN MUSCLE

If you are eating only to gain muscle (as opposed to gaining muscle and losing body fat), follow the same program described in **Appendix C**, but increase to 2600 calories for the first two weeks and to 3100 for the next two. If you are an ectomorph (a naturally skinny person who has trouble gaining weight), the caloric count may need to be as high as 3000 for the first two weeks and 3500 for the next two.

Below you will find two sample meal plans guaranteed to pack on the muscle:

WEEKS 1-2: CALORIES:MEDIUM (Approximately 2600 calories)

MEAL #1 (8:30 AM)
Carbs-54 grams; Protein 45 grams; Fats 17 grams

1 cup egg substitute	160 calories
1 cup of dry oats	300 calories
1 tablespoon flaxseed oil	130 calories

MEAL #2 (10:30 AM)
Carbs-40 grams; Protein 40 grams; Fats 8 grams

Protein Drink: 1 serving	390 calories

MEAL #3 (12:30 PM)
Carbs-50 grams; Protein 48 grams; Fats 8 grams

8 ounces chicken (weighed prior to cooking)	120 calories
1 cup salad (lettuce, tomato, carrot, cucumber, green peppers)	80 calories
10 oz baked potato	200 calories

MEAL #4 (2:30 PM)
Carbs-40 grams; Protein 40 grams; Fats 8 grams

Protein Drink: 1 serving	390 calories

MEAL #5 (4:30 PM)
Carbs-45 grams; Protein 48 grams; Fats 5 grams
Pre-Workout Meal; to be eaten at least two hours before the workout

8 oz Chicken, turkey breast or tuna (weighed prior to cooking)	240 calories
1 cup brown rice-180 calories	

6:30-7:30 PM WEIGHT TRAINING WORKOUT

MEAL #6 (7:30 PM)
Carbs-42 grams; Protein 50 grams; Fats 0 grams
Bring this meal to the gym

50 grams of protein from whey isolate product	200 calories
7 Tablespoons of cream of rice	175 calories

DAILY TOTALS
Calories: 2565; Carbohydrates: 271 grams;
Protein: 271 grams; Fats: 46 grams

WEEKS 3-4 CALORIES: HIGH (Approximately 3100 calories)

MEAL #1 (8:30 AM)
Carbs-81 grams; Protein 50 grams; Fats 20 grams

1 cup egg substitute	160 calories
1.5 cup of dry oats	450 calories
1 tablespoon flaxseed oil	130 calories

MEAL #2 (10:30 AM)
Carbs-40 grams; Protein 40 grams; Fats 8 grams

Protein Drink: 1-serving	390 calories

MEAL #3 (12:30 PM)
Carbs-50 grams; Protein 48 grams; Fats 8 grams

8 ounces chicken (weighed prior to cooking)	120 calories
1 cup salad (lettuce, tomato, carrot, cucumber, green peppers)	80 calories
10 oz baked potato	200 calories

MEAL #4 (2:30 PM)
Carbs-40 grams; Protein 40 grams; Fats 8 grams

Protein Drink: 1 serving	390 calories

MEAL #5 (4:30 PM)
Carbs 48 grams; Protein 48 grams; Fats 5 grams
Pre-Workout Meal; to be eaten at least two hours before the workout

8 oz Chicken, turkey breast or tuna (weighed prior to cooking)	240 calories
8 oz Sweet Potatoes	200 calories

6:30-7:30 PM WEIGHT TRAINING WORKOUT

MEAL #6 (7:30 PM)
Carbs-42 grams; Protein 50 grams; Fats 0 grams
Bring this meal to the gym

50 grams of protein from whey isolate product	200 calories
7 Tablespoons of cream of rice	175 calories

MEAL #7 (9:30 PM)
Carbs 18 grams; Protein 55 grams; Fats 5 grams

Protein Drink: 1 serving	390 calories

DAILY TOTALS:
Calories: 3125; Carbohydrates: 341 grams;
Protein: 316 grams; Fats: 57 grams

SUPPLEMENTS

Usually people think that supplements are the most important part of a weight-loss program. The real truth is that supplements are supplements. Supplements do not make up for improper training, bad rest habits, and a poor diet. Supplements only work when your diet and your training program are already perfect and in balance with one another.

Nutritional supplements are good because they can prevent us from having to deal with nutritional deficiencies. The increased activity levels from your new exercise program will place greater demands for vitamins and minerals on your body, which will increase the probability of you suffering a deficiency without supplementation. We cannot rely solely on foods nowadays to provide us with all the vitamins and minerals that our bodies need because the processing of foods before they get to the supermarket, the cooking process, and environmental factors rob them of many of their vitamins and minerals. If you are deficient in one or more nutrients your body may not be able to build muscle and burn fat properly. Look at supplementation as an insurance policy for avoiding possible nutritional deficiencies.

A POTENT MULTIPLE VITAMIN AND MINERAL FORMULA WITH EXTRA CALCIUM

A multiple vitamin and mineral formula with extra calcium is essential to ensure that our body operates at maximum efficiency. Why? On a very simplistic level, without vitamins and minerals it would be impossible to convert the food that we eat into hormones, tissues and energy.

Vitamins are organic compounds (produced by both animals and vegetables) whose function is to enhance the actions of proteins that cause chemical reactions such as muscle building, fat burning and energy production. There are two types of vitamins:

- **Fat-soluble vitamins-** get stored in fat and therefore if taken in excessive amounts will become toxic. These include vitamins A, D, E, and K.

- **Water-soluble vitamins-** are not stored in the body and include the B-Complex vitamins and vitamin C.

Minerals are inorganic compounds (not produced by animals or vegetables) whose main function is to assure that your brain receives the correct signals from the body, that there is a balance of fluids in the body, that muscular contractions happen and that energy production runs at peak efficiency. In addition, they are also responsible for building muscle and bones. There are two types of minerals:

- **Bulk minerals:** are named Bulk because the body needs them in great quantities (in the order of grams). They include calcium, magnesium, potassium, sodium and phosphorus.

- **Trace minerals:** are named trace because the body only needs them in minute amounts, usually in the order of micrograms. These include chromium, copper, cobalt, silicon, selenium, iron and zinc.

SOURCES:

You have to be very careful with what type of vitamin and mineral formulas you choose as some don't always contain what the labels claim and some come from such poor sources that they are not absorbed very well by the body. Some recommended formulas include the Super Spectrum Vitamin/Mineral formula, GNC's Ultra Mega, Country Life's Multi-100, and Ultra Two by Nature's Plus. Other reputable companies on the market include Twinlabs, EAS, Weider,

Labrada, Shiff, Optimum Nutrition, Advanced Nutrition, and Champion Nutrition.

QUANTITY:

Take as directed.

CHROMIUM PICOLINATE

Chromium Picolinate is a mineral that may enhance the effects of insulin, the hormone that pushes amino acids (protein) and carbohydrates into the muscle cell. As we have previously discussed, insulin is one of the most anabolic hormones in the body; it determines if the food you eat is going to be used for muscle production, energy production or fat production. When insulin is secreted in moderate levels, it aids in muscle and energy production. In excessive levels it only promotes fat storage. Chromium Picolinate may upgrade insulin's capability to produce muscle and energy by making the cells in the body more prone towards accepting this hormone. In doing so, it may help you to gain muscle and lose fat faster as insulin will now be able to deliver the desired nutrients to the muscle cell. Chromium may also keep blood sugar levels stable, thereby preventing insulin levels from going high enough to begin promoting fat storage. Again, chromium only works if we follow a proper diet. If you take chromium and continue to pig out, you will still not lose fat. As the saying goes, you can't have your cake and eat it too!

SOURCES:

All chromium picolinate produced in the market is manufactured by a company called Nutrition 21; it is sold at stores like GNC, Eckerds, Wal-mart and Walgreens.

QUANTITY:

200 mcg with the post workout meal and with breakfast on Sundays.

VITAMIN C

Vitamin C is a water-soluble vitamin that may improve your immune system and may also help you recover faster from your workouts by suppressing the amount of cortisol (hormone that breaks down muscle and aids in the accumulation of fat) that is released by your body during a workout. This is the only vitamin that may be taken in larger quantities. Because it is a water-soluble vitamin, the body will not store it. Research shows that if taken an hour before a workout (1000 mg dose) it may significantly reduce muscle soreness and speed recovery.

(Important Note: Ensure that your water intake during the day is adequate; bodyweight x 0.66 = ounces of water per day. Also ensure that you do not have a history of kidney stones as if you do, then it is not advisable that you take Vitamin C in these large quantities. As always, when in doubt, consult with your doctor).

SOURCES:

Any health food store or drug store.

QUANTITY:

1000mg (1 gram) three times a day; once with breakfast, once an hour before the workout and once with post workout meal.

MEAL REPLACEMENT POWDERS CONTAINING WHEY PROTEIN, WHEY PROTEIN POWDERS OR MEAL REPLACEMENT BARS

Because of hectic schedules, it is sometimes nearly impossible to eat the four to six perfectly balanced daily meals that are required to get in shape. Therefore, these supplements can be used as "fast foods." They are easy to prepare (if it is a protein bar then no preparation is required) and the formulas that are available on the market today are as good as a milkshake from any fast food chain (or candy bars). We recommend you use them as your mid-morning and mid-afternoon snacks if at these times you cannot have real food. If you are one of the many people that hate breakfast, you have one for breakfast as well.

PREPARATION INSTRUCTIONS:

If you purchase the full meal replacements, all you have to do is mix the packet with 16 ounces of water and you are ready to go.

If you purchase the protein powder, you'll need to mix it with at least 8 ounces of skim milk (the exact quantity of skim milk required depends on the amount of nutrients desired for the meal) and perhaps add some pieces of fruit to the drink in order to balance out the carbs (great for the post-workout meal). For non post-workout meals it is recommended that no fruits are used. Instead, ensure that a teaspoon of flaxseed oil is added in order to reduce the rate at which the simple sugars in the milk are released into the body. Remember that simple sugars are usually released too quickly into the bloodstream and if the body does not need them at that specific time, they get stored as fat. However, adding the flaxseed oil not only provides us with good essential fatty acids that we need but also slows down the simple sugar release.

If you purchase a protein bar, no preparation is required.

SOURCES:

Once again, you have to be very careful with the type of meal replacement or protein formulas you choose. Some don't contain what the label claims and some come from poor sources and are not absorbed well by the body.

Some of the best meal replacement formulas that we have seen on the market taste-wise and quality-wise are EAS Myoplex, Labrada's Lean Body, Met Rx, Biotest's Grow, Champion Nutrition's Ultramet.

One of the protein powders we recommend is Dave Draper's Bomber Blend Whey Protein, EAS Simply Protein (comes in an inexpensive 5 pound protein jug), Labrada's ProV60, ProLab's Whey Protein, and Optimum Nutrition's 100% Whey Protein (5lb jug).

Recommended protein bars include EAS Myoplex bars and Labrada's Lean Body Bars.

QUANTITY:

For Meal Replacements: 1 packet mixed with water.

For Protein Powders: 2 scoops mixed with skim milk.

For Protein Bars: 1 bar.

FISH BODY OIL CAPSULES OR FLAXSEED OIL

If you follow a very strict low-fat diet you'll find that you begin to start having trouble keeping your strength up and losing fat. It is really easy to incur a fat deficiency when your diet is really clean. Add 9 capsules of 1000 mg fish body oils a day to take care of the problem. Fish body oils may also have an anti-catabolic effect (protects muscle from breaking down) and may enhance the body's ability to burn fat by improving insulin sensitivity (the cell's ability to accept insulin). They may also help with testosterone production as well as cholesterol reduction. And if that weren't enough, they may also have antioxidant properties and protect the heart! As you can see, they are really a great supplement to add on a daily basis. If you don't like to take so many capsules, you can take three teaspoons (you can add them to either your salads or a protein shake) a day of flaxseed oil to cover your essential fatty acids needs.

SOURCES:

As far as the type of flaxseed oil we recommend, we like the refrigerated kind. If this oil is not refrigerated it loses its properties (by the way, never use this oil for cooking!). A good brand is Spectrum as this company keeps the oil refrigerated on the way to the nutrition store where it is to be sold.

You can purchase fish body oil capsules at GNC. These do not need to be kept refrigerated.

CREATINE

WHAT IS IT?

Creatine is a metabolite produced in the body composed of three amino acids: l-methionine, l-arginine and l-glycine. Approximately 95% of the concentration is found in skeletal muscle in two forms: creatine phosphate and free chemically unbound creatine. The remaining 5% of the creatine stored in the body is found in the brain, heart and testes. The body of a sedentary person metabolizes an average of 2 grams of creatine a day. Due to their high intensity training bodybuilders metabolize higher amounts. Creatine is generally found in red meats and to some extent in certain types of

fish. However it would be hard to get the amount of creatine necessary for performance enhancement as even though 2.2 lbs of red meat or tuna contain approximately between 4 to 5 grams of creatine, the compound is destroyed with cooking. Therefore, the best way to get creatine is by taking it in powder form.

HOW DOES IT WORK?

While there is still much debate as to how creatine exerts its performance enhancing benefits, it is commonly accepted that most of its effects are due to two mechanisms:

* Intra-cellular water retention.
* Creatine's ability to enhance ATP production.

Once the creatine is stored inside the muscle cell, it attracts the water surrounding each cell thereby enlarging it. This super-hydrated state causes nice side effects such as the increase of strength and the appearance of a fuller muscle. Some studies suggest that a super hydrated cell may also trigger protein synthesis and minimize catabolism.

In addition, by enhancing the body's ability to produce Adenosine Triphosphate (ATP), creatine provides for faster recovery in between sets and increased tolerance to high volume work. ATP is the compound that your muscles use for fuel whenever they contract. ATP provides its energy by releasing one of its phosphate molecules (it has three phosphate molecules). After the release of that molecule, ATP becomes ADP (Adenosine Diphosphate) as it now only has two molecules. The problem is that after 10 seconds of contraction time the ATP fuel extinguishes and in order to support further muscle contraction glycolisis (glycogen burning) has to kick in. That is fine except for the fact that as a byproduct of that mechanism lactic acid is produced.

Lactic acid is what causes the burning sensation at the end of the set. When too much lactic acid is produced, your muscle contractions stop, forcing you to stop the set. However, by taking creatine, you can extend the 10 second limit of your ATP system as creatine provides ADP the phosphate molecule that it is missing (recall that creatine is stored in the muscle as creatine phosphate). By upgrading your body's ability of regenerating ATP, you can exercise longer and harder as you will minimize your lactic acid production and you will be able to take your sets to the next level and reduce fatigue levels. More volume, strength and recovery equals more muscle (assuming nutrition and rest are dialed in).

Creatine also seems to allow for better pumps during a workout. This may be due to the fact that it possibly improves glycogen synthesis. In addition, studies have shown that creatine helps lower cholesterol and triglyceride levels.

In our own experimentation with creatine we have found that it provides all of the effects described above. As a way to prove to ourselves that these effects were not a placebo, we finally convinced one of our training partners (who was extremely skeptical about the compound) to start using it. After two weeks he noticed that for some reason he was recovering faster in between sets, had a better tolerance to high volume work and his muscles were looking fuller. He did not understand why that was happening. At such time we reminded him about the 5 grams of creatine that were being added to his post workout protein shake. While 1 subject does not provide the statistical leverage to claim that creatine will provide these effects, we are positive that provided your training, rest and nutrition are in order, you will get results out of it.

HOW TO USE IT

If you read the bottle, most companies recommend a loading phase of 20 grams for 5 days and 5-10 grams thereafter. While that is the commonly accepted way to use it, in our own experimentation we have found no benefit to loading. We have even gone as far as loading for 7 days with 40 grams a day and found no difference. As a matter of fact, my training partner only took 5 grams a day after the workout and started getting great results after only a couple of weeks. The reason for this is simple. There is only so much creatine that the body can store. Recall that the creatine is stored every time that you take it. So by taking it every day eventually you will reach the upper levels that provide the performance enhancement. After you reach that level, you could get away with just taking it on your weight training days as it takes two weeks of no use for the body's creatine levels to get back to normal.

Another issue is cycling creatine. If creatine was a supplement that loses its effectiveness as time goes by then we would recommend cycling. For example, it is beneficial to cycle fat burning supplements containing caffeine and ephedrine as the body's receptors begin to attenuate after 2 to 3 weeks of continual use. Once the body gets used to them, you need to either increase the dosage or stop their use so that the body begins to respond once again. However, that is not the way that creatine works.

Basically, creatine gets stored in your muscles and you get the effects mentioned above, period. It is really straightforward. As far as the initial weight gain that you may experience when you start taking it, whether you cycle it or not, you will get the same amount of initial weight gain as that extra weight is determined by the amount of intracellular fluid retention your muscle cells can store. The reason we say "the weight gain that you may experience" is

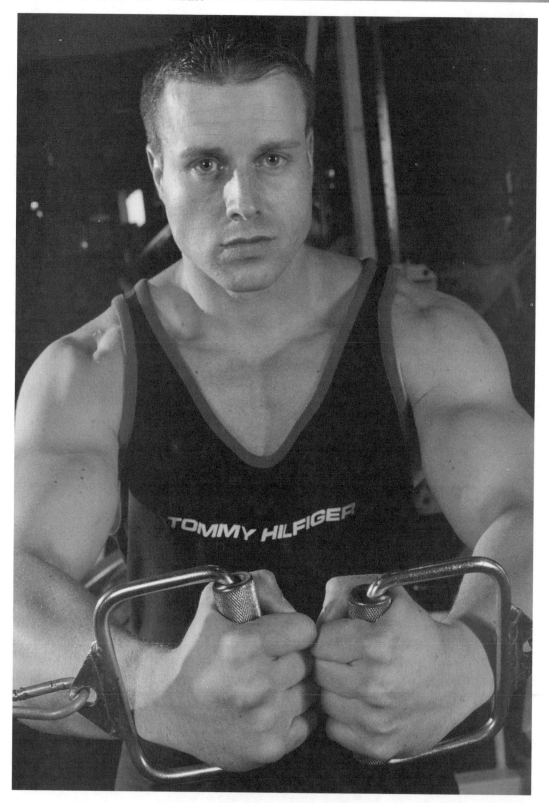

because if once you start taking it you concurrently increase the volume of your workouts and remain at the same caloric intake level you may lose fat as you gain your added muscle volume and because of that the scale might not register any weight gain (this is what happened to my training partner). However, the lack of "registered" initial weight gain by the scale does not mean that you are a "non-responder." To gauge creatine's efficacy judge the muscle appearance effects and the performance enhancement in the gym.

SIDE EFFECTS

The only adverse side effect that we have experienced in over two years of continual use is the gastric upset at the beginning of use. After a couple of weeks or so our system adapted to absorbing the powder. Other than that, we have not observed any other side effects. Keep in mind however that the liver and kidneys have to process this compound. Therefore, we would not recommend it for someone with kidney problems or liver problems. Also, even if you are completely healthy ensure more than adequate hydration levels (bodyweight x 0.66 = total ounces of water to drink per day) and if you drink coffee, add an extra 16 ounces of water for every cup that you drink over the day.

A side effect that we have read about but we are unable to quantify is that your body's production of creatine shuts down. However, after cessation of use, according to all of the literature your body's production kicks in again. No adverse effects have been documented due to the creatine shutdown created by the body.

WHAT HAPPENS IF I STOP TAKING IT?

After two weeks your creatine levels go back to normal. You will also feel weaker for about three weeks due to the fact that your ATP system is no longer enhanced. You'll also lose your enhanced recovery capabilities. In this sense, and only in this sense, creatine is like steroids. The difference is that creatine can be taken safely all of the time (opinion) while with steroids you already know the story.

However, in creatine's defense, we can also say that creatine is no different than weight training. What happens if you stop going to the gym? Will you look the same three months later?

Seriously speaking, however, since you already were lifting heavier weights while using the compound, your nervous system will remember those weights and you will be able to get back to them after 3 to 6 weeks. However, we would lower the volume when you stop taking it (go back to week 1 of the *14 Day Body Sculpting Workout*).

CREATINE AND CAFFEINE INTAKE

Years ago there were some studies suggesting that the effects of creatine were cancelled if you also had caffeine. For people like ourselves that most of the time keep caffeine at bay this does not pose any problems. However, this is not the case for people on fat burning formulas that contain caffeine. Our recommendation is that you take the caffeine (or the fat burning supplement) at a time separate from your creatine intake (take your creatine after the workout with your protein shake and take your fat burner before the workout). Also, ensure that you follow the hydration guidelines described above.

GOOD SOURCES/BAD SOURCES

We wish that we could say that all creatine supplements out there in the market are pure and effective. Unfortunately some companies out there do not take the care they should to ensure that their manufacturer is producing a quality product. Therefore use caution when purchasing a creatine product. Buy from a reputable brand like EAS, Labrada, Twinlab, Champion Nutrition, Optimum Nutrition, and Prolab. These are not the only good brands out there. However, these are the ones that we have tried and know are good. You can tell when a creatine powder is pure as it is a very fine white powder that does not get clumped up and does not look chalky. If it looks like chalk and you have to scrape it out of the container, watch out! You may be ingesting a powder that may have impurities in it. So stick to brands you know.

Also, ensure that you are buying creatine monohydrate as this is the creatine that has been used for university studies. Some companies will try to sell you creatine phosphate or creatine citrate with claims of better efficacy but such claims have not been tested.

CARBOHYDRATE LADEN CREATINE

Due to studies out there demonstrating that the body's uptake of creatine is greater when you take it in conjunction to carbs, most companies out there have been creating products that contain creatine but also high levels of sugar. My advice to you is: save your money. Buy the powder form instead as you will get much more servings of the pure compound. As long as you take it after the workout with a protein/carbohydrate rich shake I guarantee that your body will absorb the creatine with the utmost efficiency.

CONCLUSIONS

In our view the greatest advantage that creatine gives you (besides the cosmetic effect of bigger looking and fuller muscles) is that it enables you to handle more volume and recover faster in between sets by upgrading the body's capabilities to produce ATP, thereby decreasing the production of lactic acid. Therefore, in our opinion, people that will get the most benefit from creatine are those that follow a high volume, short rest in between sets type of workout (it works great for weeks 5 and 6 of the 14 Day Body Sculpting Workout). Remember that the more work that you can cram into an hour the more you'll grow (provided good cycling of volume and intensity as we have discussed in previous sections).

Even though we believe that creatine is a safe supplement, don't take our word for it if you have doubts. Do your own research and objectively review the data. If you feel creatine may be good for you, then follow the recommendations laid out in this article and provided your overall training and nutrition strategy are good, we expect that you will see results from it.

GLUTAMINE

L-Glutamine is the most abundant amino acid in muscle cells. It is released from the muscle during times of stress (such as hard weight training workouts) and dieting. This amino acid not only has been shown to be a great anti-catabolic agent (protecting the muscle from the catabolic activities of the hormone cortisol), to contribute to muscle cell volume, and to have immune system enhancing properties but also to help in the following ways:

- Regulation of protein synthesis (this is one of the ways in which steroids exert their muscle building effects).

- Accelerating glycogen synthesis after a workout.

- Sparing the use of the glycogen stored in the muscle cell (recall that the glycogen stored in the muscle cell is what gives the cell the healthy volume and firmness that you seek).

- Faster recuperation from weight training workouts.

HOW TO USE IT

Due to its anti-catabolic properties and the fact that it accelerates glycogen synthesis after a workout, glutamine is best taken 20-30 minutes after a workout with a protein shake. On days that you don't work out, just take it with your last protein shake of the day. While there is much debate amongst experts as far as dosage is concerned, we always like to remain on the conservative side. Therefore, we feel that 3 grams is a sufficient dosage. Recall that there is limited space within a muscle cell to store the glutamine so taking higher dosages will not give you better results.

As far as cycling this supplement, there is no evidence that suggests cycling would improve its efficacy.

SIDE EFFECTS

We have experienced a slight stomach discomfort during the first week of use (taking the straight powder form.) As usual, we recommend that you start with a low dosage (such as only 1 gram a day) in order to assess your tolerance. From there you can build up to the recommended dosage of 3 grams.

CONCLUSION

With the effects this supplement can provide, we wonder why more athletes don't use it. This is especially important during dieting, as a way to protect the muscle from being cannibalized by the effects of cortisol. On a final note, please remember that like any supplement you need to stick to high quality brands.

ANDROSTENDIONE

The purpose of this section is to briefly touch on the subject of Androstendione and prohormones by defining what they are and why we believe that you should stay away from them.

Prohormones are hormones that are precursors to other hormones. Androstendione is probably the most popular of all prohormones. It is a precursor to the hormone testosterone. The product is being marketed as a dietary supplement to help increase testosterone levels and produce anabolic effects similar to some of the less potent steroids. Makers of androstenedione and other prohormone supplements promote the muscle building qualities of their products due to their supposed ability to increase testosterone levels. However, this is not a true statement as such companies that make these claims are assuming that the body will convert all of the ingested Androstendione into testosterone. This is an incorrect assumption as there are many factors involved in determining how much of this prohormone will actually be converted to testosterone. Such factors include the amount of testosterone that you have in your system already, as well as the availability of the enzymes needed to make such conversion happen.

While a portion of the Androstendione that you ingest may indeed be turned into testosterone, there is a chance, depending on the chemical environment inside of your body that it may get turned into estrogen! As if this wouldn't be enough, let's remember that whenever you introduce a foreign hormone into the body, the body senses the presence of such substances and in turn, shuts down the natural production of such hormones in an attempt to keep a hormonal balance. By ingesting Androstenedione you may be short-circuiting your natural testosterone production, as the body will sense the extra amount of this hormone and then will shut down its production. Add to this the fact that some studies suggest that Androstenedione is very androgenic in nature, so side effects such as increased acne, aggressiveness and the possibility of baldness could be expected.

We wish we could tell you that this compound works as well as some companies claim it does. Since prohormones behave much like steroids, and in some cases are technically steroids, they provide many of the same problems. A study recently published in the Journal of the American Medical Association examined short and long-term effects of androstenedione supplementation in thirty young men aged 19-29 years who were not currently engaged in resistance training.

In the short-term study, 10 of the 30 men received a one-time dose of 100 mg of androstenedione. For the long-term study, the remaining 20 men performed 8 weeks of resistance training and received either 300 mg per day of androstenedione or a placebo. As expected, the androstenedione/resistance training groups did not experience a rise in free or total testosterone, nor did they experience an increase in strength. To make matters worse, test subjects in the androstenedione/resistance training group experienced a rise in HDL (high density liberal protein) cholesterol, which is the bad cholesterol, along with a rise in estrogen! So our question to you is: Why would you take something that has very similar side effects to those of anabolic steroids if you are not even going to get the so-called benefits that steroids do offer?

CONCLUSION

Our suggestion for increasing testosterone (or at least keeping it on the high range) and growth hormone in an effort to gain muscle mass is to do so by natural means such as limiting the amount of time that your weight training session lasts to an hour or less, using the correct amount of weight and rest in between sets, following a good nutrition program with the proper ratios and frequency of meals, taking 3 grams of vitamin C a day, taking 3 grams of glutamine after a workout, ensuring adequate levels of zinc and manganese in your diet, and ensuring that you get sufficient amounts of sleep. Doing this will give you measurable results in your physique and hormonal levels while at the same time improving your health and well being.

RECOMMENDED SUPPLEMENTS PROGRAM

In order of importance with the first group being the most important.

ESSENTIAL TO TAKE

- MultiVitamin/Mineral Complex taken twice daily with breakfast and protein shake after the workout (lunch if non-workout day).

- Whey Protein Powder or Meal Replacement Powder for mixing with skim milk in order to make protein shakes.

- 3 capsules of Fish Oils taken with breakfast, lunch and dinner (3 teaspoons of Flaxseed Oil if capsules are not desired)

HIGHLY RECOMMENDED (ONLY USEFUL IF YOU ARE REALLY PUSHING YOUR WORKOUTS TO THE LIMIT)

- 1 gram vitamin C taken with breakfast, lunch and dinner.

- 200mcg of Chromium Picolinate taken with protein shake after the workout.

- 2.5 grams of creatine before and after the workout.

- 3 grams of glutamine after the workout or at night-time before bed on non-workout days.

Chapter 5
Rest & Recovery

5

THE **BODY**
SCULPTING
BIBLE
FOR **MEN**

How much did you sleep last night; 5, 6, maybe 7 hours? Did you know that getting less than 6 hours a night can seriously affect your coordination, reaction time and judgment; not to mention your health?

Though the goal is to get in great shape, many of us are silently killing ourselves. With all of the stimulants now available such as high-octane coffee, ephedrine, "natural" fat burners and the like, why would we need sleep when we can simply get a "boost?" A recent article on CNN, discovered that "people who drove after being awake for 17 to 19 hours performed worse than those with a blood alcohol level of .05 percent. That's the legal limit for drunk driving in most western European countries, though most States in the U.S. set their blood alcohol limits at .1 percent and a few at .08 percent." The study revealed that 16 to 60 percent of all road accidents involved sleep deprivation.

Have you ever been in a situation where you needed to pull an "all-nighter" for school or work? We see it all the time; people bragging about not sleeping due to not having enough time in a day. Not surprisingly, nearly half of all Americans have difficulty sleeping. A growing collection of research indicates that America's sleep problems have reached epidemic proportions and may be the country's number-one health problem. Would it change your mind if you knew that those who sleep fewer than six hours a night don't live as long as those who sleep seven hours or more?

Lack of sleep can be expensive: The National Commission on Sleep Disorders estimates that sleep deprivation costs $150 billion a year in higher stress and reduced workplace productivity. Yes, most of us truly enjoy staying up late, ready to dive into the night life. We are magnetized to late night movies and late night surfing on the internet, yet did you know that we are robbing ourselves of 338 hours–two full weeks–of rest per year?

New research indicates that rest and sleep may well be the third essential component of a long and healthy life, right up there with a good diet and regular exercise! "Society is being victimized by not getting enough sleep," says David Dinges, director of experimental psychiatry at the University of Pennsylvania School of Medicine. "Our productivity, our safety, our health are at risk." The findings are far from definitive but they strongly hint that long-term sleep debt could be a factor in the national epidemics of diabetes and obesity. Research is proving that sleep deprivation could weaken the immune system, leading to colds and other infections. There is even a bit of evidence proving how the increase in breast cancer, and perhaps other cancers, could have a link to decreased sleep.

THE SLEEP CYCLE

When we deprive ourselves of sleep, there is a delicate cycle that we disrupt.

Phase One: Phase one begins as soon as the sun sets, when the pineal gland starts to release melatonin, a hormone released in the absence of light and responsible for making us sleepy. When you lay down in your bed at this time, your muscles relax, heart rate and breathing slow down, and body temperature drops. The brain also relaxes but still remains alert. If you could look at the wave patterns being generated by the brain, you would see a change from the rapid beta waves of daytime to slower alpha waves. When the alpha waves disappear, replaced by theta waves, the sleeper has tumbled into the sensory void called stage one sleep. In this stage, the sleeper is unable to sense anything.

Phase Two: Phase two occurs a moment

after phase one and in this stage the sleeper lays still for about 10 to 15 minutes.

Phase Three: After phase two is over, the sleeper falls into a deeper sleep. During this stage, the sleeper falls deeper into phase three which lasts about 5 to 15 minutes.

sleeper goes back to phase two and starts the whole process over again. These processes repeat themselves about five times during the night.

Sleep research indicates that the average sleeper will sleep approximately eight hours

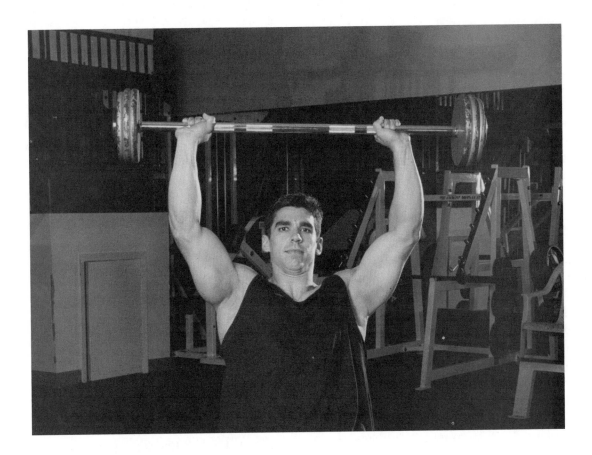

Phase Four: With a maximum of 15 minutes spent within the phase three cycle, the sleeper then falls into yet another relaxed stage called phase four, lasting a half hour or so. In stage four, the eyes move back and forth very quickly in what's called rapid eye movement, or REM. This is the point at which the first dream occurs. After this dream has ended, the

and fifteen minutes when uninterrupted. During this research, there were no alarm clocks or disturbing noises to interrupt normal sleep patterns. Eight hours and fifteen minutes is believed to be the ideal physiological amount of time that the body requires for proper sleep time.

MALADIES CAUSED BY SLEEP DEPRIVATION

The following are the maladies that according to research can be the result of consistent sleep deprivation:

Impaired glucose tolerance: Without sleep, the central nervous system becomes more active, inhibiting the pancreas from producing adequate insulin, the hormone the body needs to digest glucose. "In healthy young men with no risk factor, in one week, we had them in a pre-diabetic state," says researcher Van Cauter when referring to a study that he conducted on the effects of sleep deprivation.

Possible link to obesity: This is due to the fact that much growth hormone is secreted during the first round of deep sleep. As both men and women age, they naturally spend less time in deep sleep, which reduces growth hormone secretion. Lack of sleep at a younger age, however, could drive down growth hormone prematurely, accelerating the fat-gaining process. In addition, there is also research that indicates a lowering of the hormone testosterone as well as fat gain and muscle loss.

Increased carbohydrate cravings: Sleep deprivation negatively affects the production of a hormone called Leptin. This hormone is responsible for telling the body when it is full. However, with decreased production of this hormone, your body will crave calories (especially in the form of carbs) even though its requirements have been met. Not a good situation to be in for a dieter.

Weakened immune system: Research indicates that sleep deprivation adversely affects the white blood cell count in humans as well as the body's ability to fight infections.

Increased risk of breast cancer: Richard Stevens, a cancer researcher at the University of Connecticut Health Center, has speculated that there might be a connection between breast cancer and hormone cycles disrupted by late-night light. Melatonin, primarily secreted at night, may trigger a reduction in the body's production of estrogen. But light interferes with melatonin release (recall that the hormone is secreted in response to a lack of light), allowing estrogen levels to rise. Too much estrogen is known to promote the growth of breast cancers.

Decreased alertness and ability to focus: A recent study showed that people who were awake for up to 19 hours scored worse on performance tests and alertness scales than those with a blood-alcohol level of .08 percent–legally drunk in some states.

Hardening of the arteries: Some studies suggest that the stress imposed on the body due to lack of sleep causes a very sharp rise in cortisol levels. Such an imbalance can lead to hardening of the arteries, increasing the risk of heart attack. In addition, we also know that very high cortisol levels lead to muscle loss, increased fat storage, loss of bone mass, depression, hypertension, insulin resistance (the cells in the body lose the ability to accept insulin), and lower growth hormone and testosterone production.

Depression and irritability: Lack of sleep also causes depletion of neurotransmitters in the brain that are in charge of regulating mood. Because of this, sleep deprived people have a "shorter fuse" and also tend to get depressed more easily.

ARE YOU SLEEP DEPRIVED?

It's easy to tell if you're sleep-deprived. If you can lie down in the middle of the day and fall asleep within 10 minutes, you are sleep deprived. Catching up is basic math. For every hour, or fraction, under eight hours, you need an equal extra amount of time asleep soon after. But if you're hundreds of hours in debt, you may never pay it all off. According to recent research, 17 hours was all the catching up people could do, and it generally took three weeks. Most people probably need three times that amount of sleep!

In an earlier section, we discussed the problem of trying to get to sleep while simultaneously dealing with stress. You may refer back to page 37 to learn how to "turn off the stress light".

SLEEPING PILLS

Beware of sleeping pills! They not only tend to be addicting but people that use them find that they tend to wake up groggy. As far as melatonin supplementation, scientists are divided in opinion but most agree that the 3-milligram dose available in health food stores is too high, especially as the supplement has never been tested for safety in humans. Since we are very cautious when it comes to hormones, we would rather have you follow the guidelines below in order to ensure a good night's sleep:

- **Avoid activities that involve deep concentration** as these activities will increase adrenaline levels and will prevent the brain from achieving the state of relaxation required to achieve sleep.

- **Avoid watching disturbing shows at night on TV** as this may also increase your adrenaline levels thereby preventing you from a good night's sleep.

- **Avoid eating a large meal at night** since the digestion process will prevent you from falling asleep.

Attempt to totally relax at the same time each night. By doing so you condition the body to relax itself once the specific time that you choose comes every day. Ensure that at this time no thoughts other than relaxation and falling asleep come to your head. You need to really learn how to block all thoughts concerning work or other life issues that may be trying to get in your head. Listening to soothing music set at a low volume with the lights off can help you relax and achieve the state necessary to go to sleep.

CONCLUSION

You need 7-9 hours of sleep each night (8 being the ideal) in order for your body to run efficiently. Deprive your body of sleep and you'll have lousy fat loss and hinder your body's ability to increase lean muscle tone. Without enough sleep the body stops producing anabolic hormones (muscle producing/fat burning hormones; e.g. testosterone and growth hormone) and starts increasing the production of catabolic hormones (muscle destroying/fat depositing hormones e.g. cortisol). So, to make matters worse, you'll also lose muscle, which lowers your metabolism. In addition, you will lack the energy and focus to get through your workouts, which will surely lead to overtraining. To top it off, research indicates that lack of sleep creates cravings and binges in addition to hardening of the arteries, which leads to heart attacks. In short: **turn off the TV, relax and hit the sack!**

Part 3
Body Sculpting Exercises

Learning proper exercise technique is the backbone of every fitness program. If you train improperly you will not stimulate the intended muscle, and will risk major injury as well as receive little or no results. When you learn to use proper exercise technique you will receive twice the results in half the time, guaranteed! I see people in the gym day in and day out who have no idea how to properly train their muscles. Some of them are professional bodybuilders, some are professional athletes, and some are even certified fitness trainers. Unfortunately, the ones who really suffer the most are people like you who rely on these role models for wisdom and guidance. We will show you the proper exercise technique to use for optimal results. Just remember to utilize your newfound knowledge. Like the old saying, "Feed a man a fish and he'll eat for a day, teach a man to fish and he'll eat for a lifetime." We expect the same of you. We don't want you to read this book once and then forget everything you've learned. We want you to learn and utilize that knowledge to achieve astounding results.

Applying proper exercise form and technique is, without doubt, the most important component of any fitness program. Without it, many, many setbacks will occur. First, the musculature you intend to exercise will not be stimulated as efficiently as possible. Exercise should not be focused around just lifting barbells and weights. It shouldn't just be about how much you can lift. Optimum fitness is about the quality of exercise, the quality of your form and how you maintain that form, especially during heavier lifting. Proper exercise technique coupled with the Zone-Tone principle will bring you the most astonishing results with the minimum amount of sets. Why? Because as we have already discussed, one properly executed set is equivalent to five sets of "just going through the motions" type of exercise. It comes down to this; if you want to get the most out of your workout, keep the intensity high without sacrificing proper form. Neglecting to focus on proper form equals no results, while practicing perfect proper form equals incredible results quickly!

Chapter 6
Legs

We decided to start the exercise description part of this book by discussing leg exercises. There are many reasons for this.

First of all, many guys just want to go to the gym and workout their upper bodies. These guys claim that their legs are 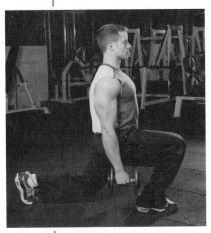"fine". This attitude is OK if what you want to do is end up looking like a light bulb with two pencils for legs. Don't you guys know that the best bodies have tight looking legs accompanied with a nice firm behind? Besides, do you realize how much upper body growth you are missing out on if you decide not to work out the legs? The reason for this is because hard leg exercises, like the squat, stimulate more testosterone and growth hormone than any other exercises out there. Besides, there are very few lifts that require the use of all of the muscles in the body the way that the back squat does.

Now that you realize how important leg exercises are, you're ready to learn how to perform the king of all exercises: the Barbell Squat.

6

THE BODY SCULPTING BIBLE FOR MEN

Barbell Squat

One of the best exercises you can do to build strong, ripped legs is the squat. This exercise is also known to provide beneficial results to the whole body because you use several body muscles to synergistically join forces and execute the lift.

It will primarily help develop the quadriceps muscles, and secondarily stimulate the hamstring muscles, the gluteal muscles, and the calves. However, it also will incorporate virtually all the body's major muscle groups in one way or another.

PROPER ALIGNMENT

1. Place a bar on either a squat safety rack or in a power cage, making sure you have the safety bars set just about even with the height of your thighs when they are parallel to the floor.

2. Walk up to the bar and place your shoulders comfortably underneath it, making sure that the bar rests on the trapezoid muscles and not on the first and second cervical vertebrae. A shoulder pad is good to use. You can find them at most sporting good stores, or simply use a rolled up towel!

3. Position your hands on the bar with a double shoulder width grip.

4. Before lifting up the bar, either take a ready stance, making sure your body is properly aligned or, as we recommend, slowly step backwards with the weight already on your shoulders. This allows more room for the movement. If you are nervous about stepping backwards with the weight, you can always use the first option; or maybe you should re-evaluate how much weight you will be lifting. Whenever you feel nervous, be smart and consider either going a little lighter or having a qualified spotter assist you with the lift. Also, please don't just take someone's word for being a good spotter. Either ask reliable sources for someone who is qualified, or look around for someone whom you observe as a good spotter.

5. Always align your body, starting from the bottom and moving to the top:

First, align your feet, making sure they are about shoulder width apart with a slight outward angle.

Next, slightly bend your knees to reduce undue stress from the lower back area.

Position your knees so that they are pointing directly in front of you.

Slightly contract the muscles of your lower back and the muscles of your abdominal section. This will ensure that you stay in proper alignment throughout the movement.

Stick out your chest while simultaneously squeezing your shoulder blades together. This helps to set the upper body in its proper position.

Finally, keep your head level at all times. Make sure your head and your eyes do not drop down or wander upward excessively as this is an easy way to lose your balance and fall. we would rather you look slightly above level rather than below as looking below level can greatly affect your equilibrium and jeopardize your safety.

TECHNIQUE AND FORM

Once you think you have properly aligned yourself, repeat the alignment steps starting from the bottom and moving up. Once you have secured your alignment, prepare to inhale as you begin your descent downward. As you execute the movement, keep the following points in mind:

1. As you are squatting downward, it is very important that at no time throughout the movement do your knees go forward beyond your toes. This puts way too much pressure on the knees, and can seriously damage them. Here is a technique that will help keep this from happening: As you begin your descent, mimic the motion and alignment of sitting in a chair. Make sure you keep your back as straight as possible. This motion will naturally help you to utilize the proper form.

2. Make sure you don't let your thighs go below parallel as you could injure your lower back and knees.

3. As you reach parallel or just above it, begin to exhale and press off your feet, distributing the weight through the heel while pressing upward. You must concentrate on keeping and holding proper alignment throughout the movement.

4. As you reach the top of the movement, make sure you do not lock out your knees since this will put too much stress on the knee joint. If at any time during the movement you should feel or notice yourself getting sloppy or not retaining the proper alignment, stop immediately! Never jeopardize your safety with bad form.

5. When you've done the desired amount of reps, walk the bar back into the rack and place it down.

Barbell Squat

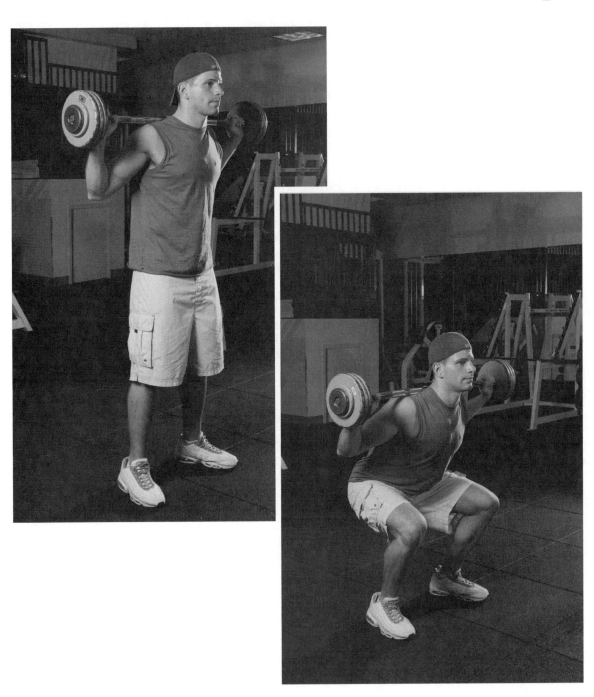

Dumbbell Squat

This exercise emphasizes the same muscles as the barbell squats. Performing the exercise with dumbbells, however, places less stress on the lower back. Use this variation if all you have available is a pair of dumbbells or if you have had lower back injuries.

PROPER ALIGNMENT:

1. Hold a dumbbell in each hand with arms extended down and palms facing your body.

2. Align your body from the bottom up by first taking a shoulder-width stance.

3. Slightly bend your knees and avoid locking them during this exercise.

4. Contract your abdominal muscles to help support and sustain your posture during the exercise.

5. Stick your chest out and simultaneously bring your shoulder blades back, keeping them there throughout the movement.

6. Keep your head level at all times, making sure your head or your eyes do not drop down, or excessively wander upward. This is an easy way to lose your balance and fall. It is preferable to look slightly above level rather than below because looking below level can greatly affect your equilibrium and jeopardize your safety.

7. If you feel unstable, you may put small 2 1/2 pound plates under each heel for stability.

TECHNIQUE AND FORM:

1. When you think you have properly aligned yourself, repeat the alignment steps starting from the bottom and moving up. Once you have secured your alignment, prepare to inhale as you begin your descent.

2. As you are squatting downward, it is very important that at no time throughout the movement your knees go forward beyond your toes. This puts way too much pressure on the knees and can seriously damage them. Here is a technique that will help prevent this from happening: As you begin your descent, mimic the motion and alignment of sitting in a chair. Make sure you keep your back as straight as possible. This motion will naturally help you to utilize the proper form.

3. Make sure you don't let your thighs go below parallel as you could injure your lower back; and this can also push the knees past the toes, once again leading to injury.

4. As you reach parallel or just above it, begin to exhale and press off your feet, distributing the weight through the heel while pressing upward.

Concentrate on keeping and holding proper alignment throughout the movement.

5. As you reach the top of the movement, make sure you do not lock out your knees since it will put too much stress on the knee joint. If at any time during the movement you should feel or notice yourself getting sloppy or not retaining the proper alignment, stop immediately! Never jeopardize your safety with bad form!

6. When you've done your desired amount of reps, simply squat down once again and place the dumbbells on the floor or place them back on the dumbbell rack. Never bend over to either pick up or place the dumbbells down. Doing this can injure your lower back area.

Dumbbell Squat

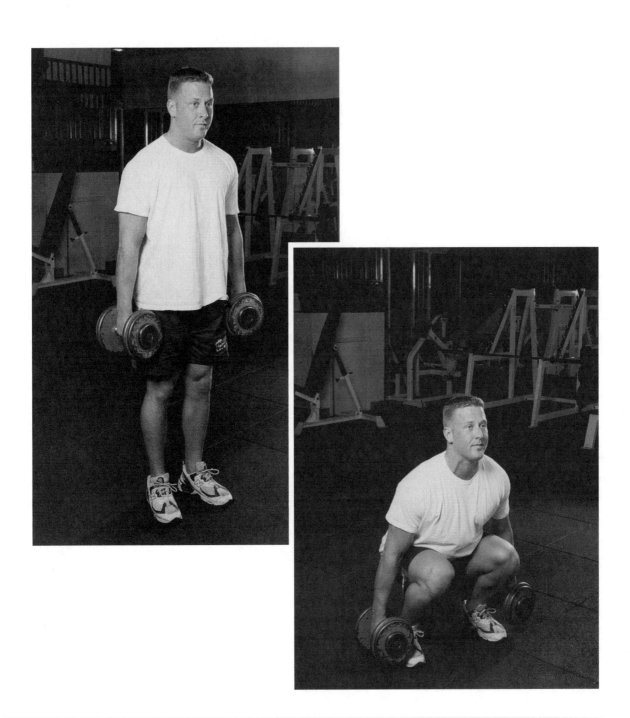

Ballet Squat

This exercise is to be performed the same way as the barbell or dumbbell versions described above with the exception that your foot stance will be wider than shoulder width. This variation will yield a stronger emphasis on the inner quads. Some guys are afraid that a wide stance will give them a big butt and hips. This is not true. A wide-stance squat can actually help shape the quadriceps and the inner thighs. You must make sure though that you don't have too wide a stance. An overly wide stance can cause knee problems and possibly generate some rather painful groin pulls. A good stance is about 1-1/2 times shoulder width with the toes pointed outward at a minimum of 25-30 degrees. No matter how wide your stance, your ankles should always remain in line with your knees. A good indication that a stance is too wide is when the ankles are outside of the knees in the bottom position of a squat. While you are discovering the width of stance best suited for you, don't worry about the amount of weight to use. Instead concentrate on your overall technique and form with your adjusted stance.

PROPER ALIGNMENT

1. Hold a dumbbell in each hand with arms extended down and palms facing your body or a barbell on your back with your arms holding the barbell in place.

2. Align your body from the bottom up by first taking a shoulder-width stance.

3. Slightly bend your knees and avoid locking out your knees anytime during this exercise.

4. Contract your abdominal muscles to help support and sustain your posture during exercise.

5. Stick your chest out and simultaneously bring your shoulder blades back, keeping them there throughout the movement.

6. Keep your head level at all times. Make sure your head and your eyes do not drop down or wander upward excessively as this is an easy way to lose your balance and fall. We would rather you look slightly above level, rather than below, as looking below level can greatly effect your equilibrium and jeopardize your safety.

7. If you feel unstable, you may put small 2 1/2 pound plates under each heel for stability.

TECHNIQUE AND FORM

1. When you think you have properly aligned yourself, repeat the alignment steps, starting from the bottom and moving up. Once you have secured your alignment, prepare to inhale as you begin your descent.

2. As you are squatting downward, it is very important that at no time throughout the movement your knees go forward beyond your toes. This puts way too much pressure on the knees, and can seriously damage them. Here is a technique that will help keep this from happening: As you begin your descent, mimic the motion and alignment of sitting in a chair. Make sure you keep your back as straight as possible. This motion will naturally help you to utilize the proper form.

3. Make sure you don't let your thighs go below parallel since you could injure your lower back; this can also push the knees past the toes, once again leading to injury.

4. As you reach parallel or just above it, begin to exhale and press off your feet distributing the weight throughout the heel while pressing upward. You must concentrate on keeping and holding proper alignment throughout the movement.

5. As you reach the top of the movement, make sure you do not lock out your knees since it will put to much stress on the knee joint. If at any time during the movement you should feel or notice yourself getting sloppy or not retaining the proper alignment, stop immediately! Never jeopardize your safety with bad form!

6. When you've done your desired amount of reps, simply walk the bar back to the rack. Or, if using dumbbells, squat down once again and place them on the floor or back on the dumbbell rack. Never bend over to either pick up or place the dumbbells down. Doing this can most definitely injure your lower back area.

Ballet Squat

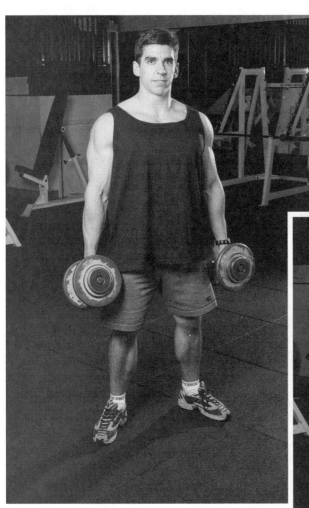

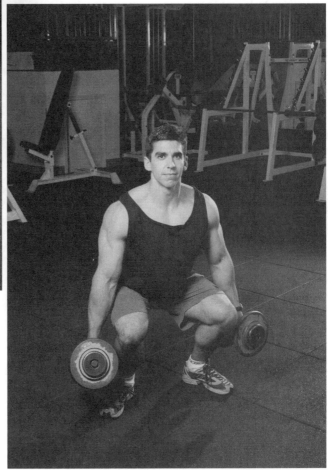

Dumbbell Lunge

This exercise is an excellent movement for all of the muscles in the legs. It primarily stresses the buttocks, hamstrings and quads with a secondary emphasis on the calves. This movement can also be performed with a barbell on the back. The barbell variation, however, places more stress on the lower back. If you choose to use a barbell, use the same steps described below in order to perform the movement.

Lunges are a fantastic leg exercise for both men and women. Due to the fact that only one leg is used at a time, lunges require a balancing act. In order to maintain balance the body needs to recruit as many auxiliary fibers as possible. What this means to you is more muscle stimulation per repetition. In addition, lunges can be used to stimulate the hamstrings muscles or the quadriceps muscles by varying how far away you place your foot. If when you step forward you place your foot closer to your body, you will primarily stimulate the quadriceps. If when you step forward you place your foot farther away from your body, you will primarily stimulate the hamstrings. (Note: In no case, as you'll see in the exercise description, should your knee go past your toes.)

PROPER ALIGNMENT:

1. Hold a dumbbell in each hand with arms extended down and palms facing your body.

2. Align your body from the bottom up, first taking a stance with the feet together, and the toes pointing straight ahead.

3. Keep your knees slightly bent to avoid any stress from locking the knee joint.

4. Slightly contract the abdominal muscles.

5. Stick the chest out while simultaneously bringing the shoulder blades back, keeping them there throughout the movement.

6. Keep your head level at all times, making sure your head or your eyes do not drop down or excessively wander upward.

TECHNIQUE AND FORM:

1. Step forward with your right foot.

2. Bend at the knee making sure you descend slowly and in control.

3. As your knee bends and your hips are lowering, lower yourself only until your left knee is about two inches from the ground and then stop.

4. When you step forward at the beginning of the movement, make sure that the knee does not go past the toes when you are in the bent-knee position with your left knee two inches from the ground.

5. Begin to reverse the movement by pressing off the right foot only. You may naturally want to use the left knee to assist in pushing back up, but do not let this happen. The objective is to fully isolate the right leg muscles and use the left leg only as a balancing tool, sort of like the rudder on a boat.

6. Make sure you do not use momentum as you push off with the right leg to return. This will totally inhibit the stimulation of the leg muscles.

7. Return to the start position but do not rest. Switch legs and repeat the same movement making sure to maintain the alignment and posture throughout the movement.

Dumbbell Lunge

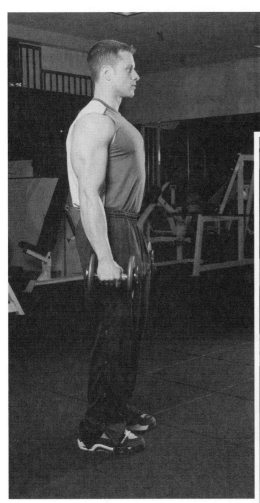

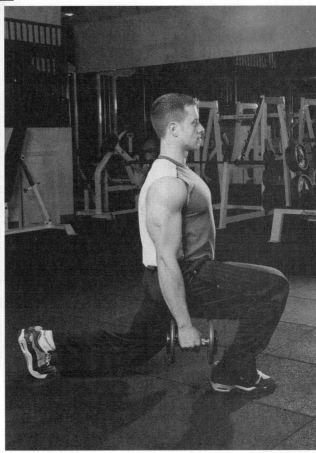

Leg Press

The leg press machine is a great exercise for the legs. It can be used in place of the traditional barbell squat for people that suffer from lower back pain, as a rehabilitation exercise (especially if only using one leg at a time) or to just supplement your leg routine.

There are two ways to perform this exercise: one leg at a time or both legs at the same time. In this book we will discuss the more common two-legged version. However, the execution for the exercise remains the same for both versions.

PROPER ALIGNMENT

1. Sit on machine with your back on the padded support and align your feet evenly on the platform. The height placement of your feet on the platform will zone in on different areas of the quadriceps. The higher your foot placement on the platform the less intense the quad contraction and the less knee involvement.

The lower your foot placement on the platform, the more intense the quad contraction will be; but you will put a lot of stress and shear force on the knees.

2. Make sure that your back and head are kept flush against the back pad and that you are seated securely in the seat.

3. Take hold of the release lever handles and disengage the lock pins.

TECHNIQUE & FORM

1. Immediately take hold of the secured handles, which are usually located to the sides of you. If the handles are placed in an awkward position, you can also take hold of the seat edge. This can help take some stress off the lower back.

2. With the feet spaced evenly apart and flat upon the platform, slowly lower the sled towards you.

3. Once again, do not grip the handles too tightly.

4. Let the sled come down to a point just before your thighs would touch your chest. Depending on your condition, you might not want to bring the sled this low. Monitor your individual situation. Too many trainees don't allow the sled to go deep enough to sustain any type of quad muscle

involvement, and they'll pack on the weights. Lighten the weight and tone!

5. When you have reached the bottom portion of the exercise, return back to the starting position by slowly pushing the platform evenly with both feet. Do not lock your knees! This could injure your knees and will also take the resistance off of the quads, distributing it directly to the knee joints.

Leg Press

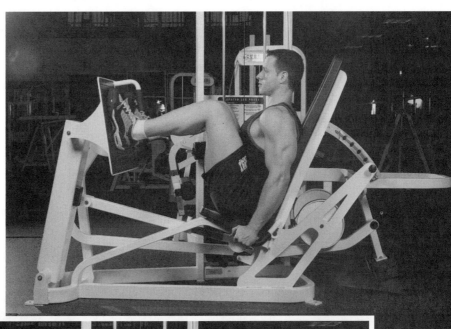

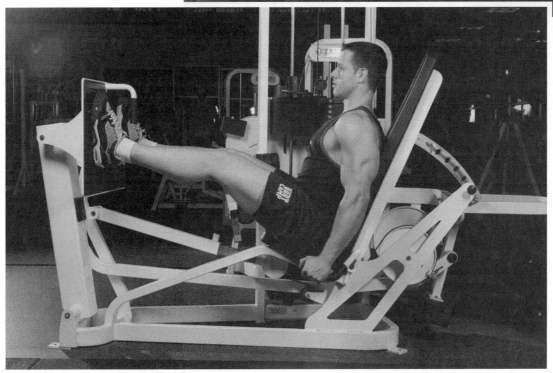

Leg Extension

The leg extension is an excellent isolation exercise that really targets the quadriceps muscles located on the front of the thigh. It also helps strengthen the knee, which is a commonly injured area. The leg extension is recommended by most physical therapists as a good tool for knee rehabilitation. The key to the effectiveness and safety of this exercise is to choose a machine whose starting position allows your toes to be right in front of your knees and to focus on contracting the thigh muscle (as opposed to lifting heavy) as you lift the weight. Focusing on lifting heavy weights will cause knee damage, especially if you are using a machine in which your toes start behind your knees (in this case the upper leg and the lower leg will be at an angle that is below 90-degrees).

There are two ways to perform this exercise: one leg at a time (in which case you will not be able to use as much weight) or both legs at the same time. In this book we will discuss the more common two-legged version. However, the execution for the exercise remains the same for both versions.

PROPER ALIGNMENT:

1. Seat yourself on the machine and position the back pad so that you are sitting totally upright.

2. The back of your knees must be pressed flush against the front of the seat, which will help you avoid a potential knee injury caused by allowing the knee to hang over the seat without support. Doing this will give the needed support to your knees. You also want to make sure that the axis of the knees are in line with the machine axis, helping to set up the proper alignment (biomechanics) of the knee and direct the maximum resistance to the quadriceps. In addition, as discussed previously, ensure that the starting position allows the toes to be in front of the knees and that the upper leg and lower leg create a 90-degree angle.

3. Adjust the shin roller pad against the lowest point of the shin to help optimize the shin as a lever and the knee as the fulcrum. This will again help to direct the majority of the resistance to the thigh muscles. Before you begin the exercise, lightly grip the handles provided or grab the front of the seat on each side of your legs.

TECHNIQUE AND FORM:

1. Begin the exercise with your legs totally relaxed and your shins behind the roller pad positioned at the bottom.

2. Isometrically contract the quad muscles and slowly begin to lift the weight by lifting the roller pad with the shins.

3. As you extend upward, stay in control by allowing the quad muscles to lift the weight. Do not use momentum or leverage. This is a very easy exercise to cheat on by using quick bursts of momentum at the bottom of the movement, or by leaning back and using leverage to lift the weight.

4. As you reach the point of full extension, when the part of your leg below your knee is extended and as close as possible to being in a direct line with your upper thigh, focus only on fully contracting the quad muscles. Sometimes people have the tendency to go through the exercise motions without consciously contracting the muscles that are supposed to be lifting the weight. As long as you make a great effort to squeeze or contract the quad muscle fully at the top of full extension, you will be taking full advantage of the exercise.

5. Make sure that once you get to the fully extended position of the exercise, you don't just let the leg drop but slowly return back to the beginning of the movement.

6. As you reach the bottom, do not rest! Slowly and smoothly lift the roller pad with your shins back to full extension. Always make sure that you are going through the full range of motion for these exercises as doing so will provide the maximum muscular development.

Leg Extension

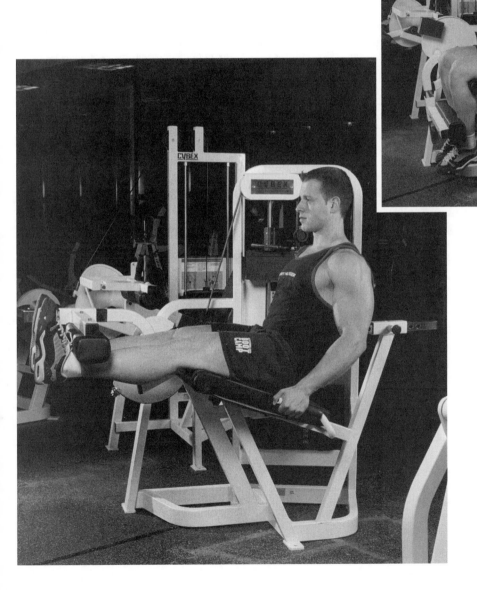

Lying Leg Curl

The lying leg curl is an exercise that focuses on the hamstrings located on the back of the upper leg. It also affects the gluteal muscles and the muscles of the lower back (erector spinae). Again, form over weight is crucial! It is very easy to pull a hamstring if you are using heavy weights and jerking the weights!

There are two ways to perform this exercise: one leg at a time or both legs at the same time. In this book we will discuss the more common two-legged version. However, the execution for the exercise remains the same for both versions.

PROPER ALIGNMENT:

There are several machines for training the hamstring muscles, but we recommend the lying leg curl machine. If you prefer, you may use the seated leg curl machine instead. No matter which machine you choose, the alignment will basically be the same.

1. Position yourself on the machine and, as always, begin the alignment of your body starting with your feet.

2. Lock your pelvis into place by contracting your abdominal muscles.

3. Try to focus only on the hamstring muscles.

4. When you're lying down, relax your upper body. (Allowing your body to stay tense during the exercise will only negatively affect hamstring stimulation.) If you like, you can hold on to the set of handles, which are usually supplied. Just make sure you do so with a very light grip. Squeezing too hard can change the focus of resistance in the hamstring muscles, causing this exercise to be less beneficial. Holding too tight can also cause leverage to do the work for you instead of working the muscle. Remember, don't sell yourself short trying to find the easy way of exercising. You are here to work, not to make things easy. Besides, work is what produces results, not the alternative.

5. Relax your neck and head. If you choose the seated leg curl machine, you should follow the same form; that is, space your feet evenly.

6. Keep your knees pointed directly in front of you throughout the movement.

7. Contract your abdominal muscles and relax your upper body, neck and head.

TECHNIQUE AND FORM:

1. As you begin the movement, contract the hamstrings before actually moving as this will help to focus the resistance on the hamstring muscles and better stimulate the those muscles.

2. Drive your heels to your butt, while pointing (this is very important) your toes toward your knees ("flexing your feet"). It will be the same whether sitting or lying down. Pointing your toes towards your knees helps to better isolate the hamstring muscles. Refer to pictures on showing the relaxed feet and the flexed feet positions.

3. When you reach your butt, try to hold that position for a count of two seconds. This will help increase the intensity of the exercise; and once again, better stimulate the hamstring muscles.

As you descend, do so with a slow, controlled movement. When you reach the starting position, without rest, slowly and smoothly change directions, moving upward once again. Following these guidelines will ensure your safety and greater results.

RELAXED

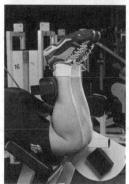

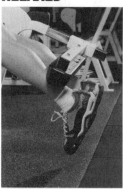

Lying Leg Curl

FLEXED

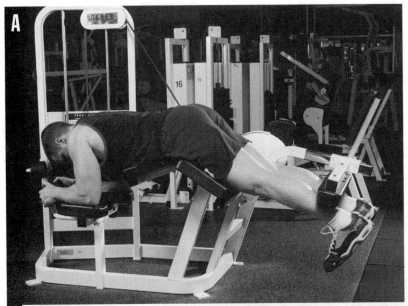

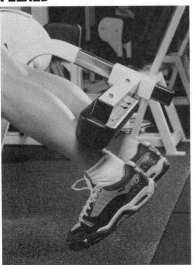

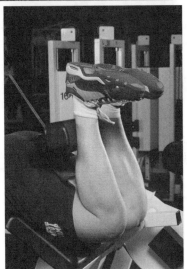

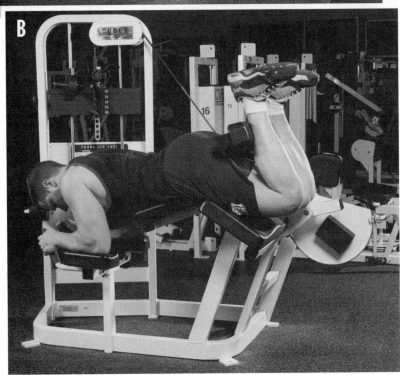

Seated Leg Curl

This variation of the leg curl is great for simply adding variety to your hamstring training and also for preventing problems in some injury-prone areas such as the lower back. If you suffer from lower back problems and have access to this machine, feel free to use it. However, like any machine, the key is to focus on the form and not add weight haphazardly. Any machine will injure you if you use too much weight with improper form.

PROPER ALIGNMENT

1. Position yourself on the seated leg curl machine with your shins placed against the roller pads.

2. Make sure to align your knees with the axis of the rotating pivot joint of the machine.

3. Position the back pad forward or backward for the proper alignment of your knees with the axis.

4. Loosely place your hands on the handles that are provided on the side of the machine.

5. Keep your head relaxed and your back flat against the back pad at all times during the exercise.

TECHNIQUE AND FORM

1. Keeping your legs locked in place from your knee to your hip, bend your knees and curl the bottom portion of your legs down as far as you can go.

2. Hold for a brief second while simultaneously contracting (flexing) your hamstrings.

3. Slowly return to the starting position in a slow, controlled manner.

4. You may hold onto the handles located on the side of the seat to keep your body locked in place during the exercise-just don't squeeze the handles too hard as it may take away from the focus on the hamstrings.

5. Keep your head straight and avoid looking down during the exercise. Keeping your head in a neutral position will help maintain your overall balance.

6. Don't let your back round. Keeping it straight will help take pressure off your lower back.

Seated Leg Curl

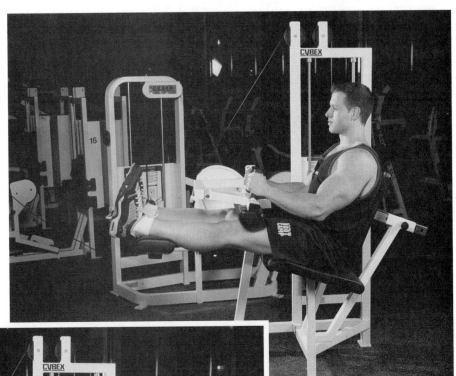

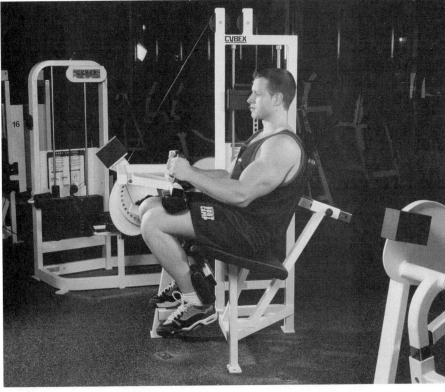

Standing Leg Curl

This variation of the leg curl is a great way to both isolate the hamstring muscles and to focus on possible imbalances between the two legs. It is basically the equivalent of performing a barbell curl but for the leg biceps instead. You can do a great variation of this exercise at home by simply strapping on some ankle weights and holding on to a stationary object for stability. You can also use elastic cables strapped to a stationary object on one end and to your ankle on the other end. Use this exercise in lieu of the stiff legged deadlifts if you suffer from lower back problems.

PROPER ALIGNMENT

1. Stand next to the lever arm of the machine so that it is to the right of your leg.

2. Hook your right heel under the roller pad attached to the lever arm.

3. The type of machine you have access to will either allow you to kneel upon the knee rest with your left leg or stand with your left leg on a platform, which will keep your body elevated for your right leg to clear the platform when performing the exercise movement.

TECHNIQUE AND FORM

1. Keeping your upper leg from your knee to your hip securely in place, curl your right leg up as high as it will go, using your hamstring muscle.

2. At the top, contract your hamstring muscle as hard as you can and hold for one second.

3. Slowly return to the bottom in a controlled and smooth motion.

4. Perform the determined reps for one leg, switch legs and do the same number of reps for the other leg.

5. Make sure not to jerk or allow momentum to assist you with the exercise.

Standing Leg Curl

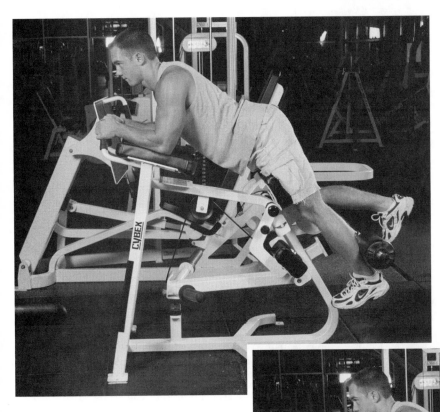

Stiff-Legged Deadlift

The stiff-legged deadlift is a very good exercise for the hamstring muscles (located between your butt and knees) and the lower back "erector" muscles provided that:

You concentrate on perfect form and avoid using heavy weights.

You do not suffer from lower back problems.

You avoid going to total muscle failure.

You can do this exercise either with a barbell or while holding two dumbbells. If you have a lower back injury, we advise that you don't do this exercise. Although it is a fantastic exercise to help strengthen the lower back, if you already have a lower back injury, it can do more harm than good. If this is the case, use the standing leg curl exercise (with either a machine, ankle weights or elastic cables) instead.

PROPER ALIGNMENT:

1. First, choose a weight for your barbell or dumbbells, making sure that the weight is light enough to practice perfect form.

2. Position your feet shoulder width apart, pointing straight ahead at all times during the movement.

3. Position your hands on the barbell with a grip wider than your feet position. Your hands positioned slightly outside your foot stance should be adequate.

4. Stand up straight and hold the barbell across your thighs or the dumbbells at your side with your palms facing toward your legs.

5. The object here is to keep your legs completely straight, staying locked at the knee joints and bending forward at the waist. It is very, very important to make sure you keep your back completely straight while bending forward. I recommend that as you bend down, you keep your head and eyes looking straight ahead and level. If you look down at the ground, you will be very likely to hyper-flex your spine and cause a lower back injury.

TECHNIQUE AND FORM

Before you begin the exercise and throughout the execution, you must direct all of your focus to the hamstring muscles of the rear thigh, to help activate them even more. "Put your mind in the muscle!" When you return to the starting top position of the exercise, focus on the erector muscles of the lower back by slightly arching the spine and sticking the chest out, contracting those lower back muscles.

1. With your body straight, legs locked and arms hanging down, begin the exercise by bending over at the waist.

2. Remember to look straight ahead as you bend over. Your eyes must be looking level with your body as you reach parallel to the floor.

3. As you bend over, concentrate on the hamstring muscles of the thigh and make sure your back is maintained in a straight position as you lower yourself.

4. As you reach a point when your torso is parallel to the floor and the bar or dumbbells are fairly close to touching the floor, slowly and without rest begin lifting your body back up from

the waist, concentrating on focusing all of the work to the hamstring muscles of the thigh. Do not use any momentum during this movement, especially at this position! You will really feel the hamstring muscles contract in the lower position as you slowly change directions and begin your way upward.

5. Keep your head and eyes looking straight ahead as you return to the standing position.

6. As you return to the start position, really contract your hamstring muscles, but don't stop there. As you stand straight up, stick your chest way out and slightly arch your spine while you contract the muscles of the lower back.

7. Hold that position for only one second, then slowly and smoothly begin lowering your body again, maintaining the same exact form as when you began the exercise.

Stiff-Legged Deadlift

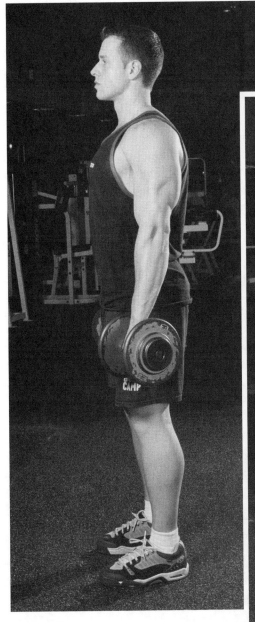

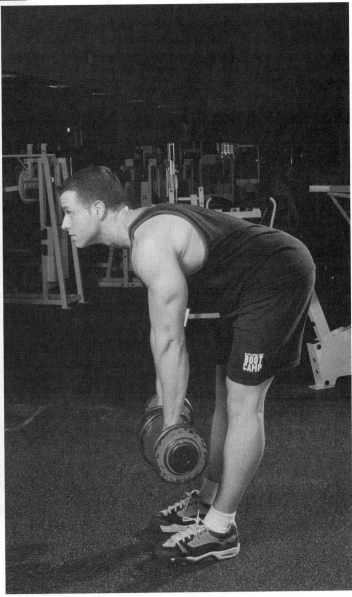

Calf Raises

The calf muscles may be thought of as just a small part of the large spectrum of body parts, but having good calf development can mean the difference between having a great body versus having an assymetrical weak looking one. The calves are one of the most eye-catching areas of the body, and are often associated with how fit a person really is. The calves, abdominals and shoulder muscles are three areas of the body that seem to work with each other. If one of the three is out of balance with the others, it can have a terrible effect on the overall appearance of your body. On the other hand, if all three body parts are in sync with each other, your body will look like a symmetrical whole.

The calf muscles are very stubborn and they won't respond to training unless you train them correctly. Besides needing different angles of training with proper technique and form, they need a lot of weight and repetitions in order to grow. If you think about how much work your calves do every day with just your normal routine (walking, running, sitting down, standing up, etc.), and take into account that these activities are done with your full body weight; you can see why your calf muscles would require special training to grow. The calf muscles have adapted to the rigors of everyday life. You must introduce them to training that they are not used to—heavy weight with high repetitions! This will shock them, and they will now be forced to adapt to the new training by growing!

In this program, we will discuss four exercises that will help you tremendously in reshaping your calf muscles. The standing calf raise, calf press and donkey calf raise will primarily help develop mass in the bulk of the muscle (gastrocnemius muscle) and secondarily stimulate the soleus muscles (lower and outer portions of the calf); and the seated calf raise will primarily target the soleus muscles. Of crucial importance when perfoming calf exercises is to focus on stretching the muscle at the bottom of the movement and contracting the muscle at the top. Typically, when we train calves, we like to spend a second in the stretched (bottom) position and a second or two in the contracted (top) position.

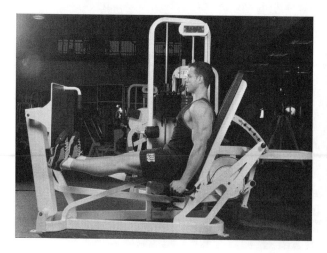 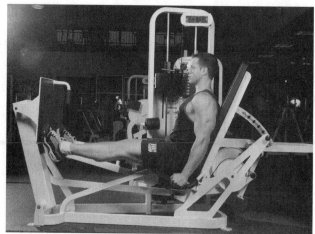

STANDING CALF RAISE

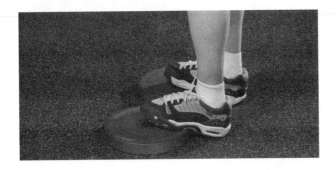 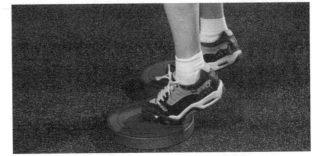

CALF PRESS

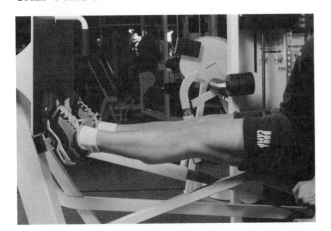 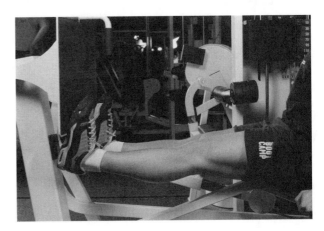

SEATED CALF RAISE

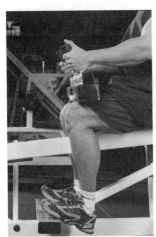 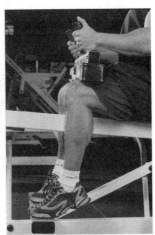

DONKEY CALF RAISE

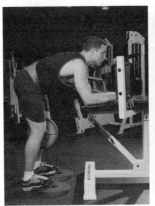 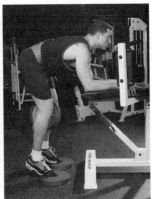

Standing Calf Raise

(Using A Machine, Barbell Or Dumbbells)

The standing calf raise machine is a great tool for building quality calves. If you don't have access to a calf raise machine, you may use a pair of dumbbells instead to hold at your sides. Of course, you'll want to get yourself a pair of dumbbells that you can add extra weight to.

There are two ways to perform this exercise: one leg at a time (holding yourself to a stationary object if using dumbbells) or both legs at the same time. For this exercise, you can use dumbbells, barbells or a machine. In this book we will discuss the more common two-legged version in a machine. However, the execution for the exercise remains the same for all versions.

PROPER ALIGNMENT

For the machine:

1. Set the weight to a resistance you can handle while practicing perfect form.

2. Step on the platform and take hold of the grip bars on the sides of the shoulder harness.

3. With your feet pointing straight ahead, place your toes and the balls of your feet on the platform.

4. Set the shoulder pads so they will be slightly lower than your shoulders while you are in this position.

5. Bend at the knees and position your shoulders underneath the shoulder pads comfortably.

6. Stand up straight so that your shoulders lift the shoulder pads, which will lift the weight plates up.

7. Keep your knees pointing straight ahead and keep them bent very slightly during the exercise. The bent-knee position can help stretch the calves in the lower position and will save your lower back in the upper position.

8. Make sure to keep your body straight during the exercise. Be careful not to bend at the waist during any portion of the movement or hyperextend your back at the top of the movement. Doing either of these can injure your back.

9. Stick your chest out and keep your shoulders squared at all times during the exercise.

10. Keep your head straight and level and look straight ahead at all times.

For dumbbells:

1. First, pick up the dumbbells and stand in front of a platform, which should be about 1 inch high.

2. Step onto the platform and position your feet a couple of inches apart.

3. Bring the dumbbells to the sides of your body, with your palms facing each other.

4. Place your toes and the balls of your feet on the platform.

5. Keep your knees pointing straight ahead and keep them bent very slightly during the exercise as the bent knee position can help stretch the calves in the lower position and will save your lower back in the upper position.

6. You must make sure to keep your body straight during the exercise. Be careful not to bend at the waist during any portion of the movement or hyperextend your back at the top of the movement. Doing either of these can injure your back.

7. Stick your chest out and keep your shoulders squared at all times during the exercise.

8. Keep your head straight and level and look straight ahead at all times.

TECHNIQUE AND FORM

The technique and form will be the same for both the standing machine and the standing dumbbell raise.

1. Keeping your body as straight as possible, lower your heels toward the floor and slowly bring the calves to a full stretch.

2. Hold this position for a count of 1 second.

3. From this position, without momentum, push off the balls of your feet and come up on to your tiptoes, pushing as high off the toes as possible. Contract the calves as hard as you possibly can and concentrate all of your efforts on doing so. Hold this position for a 1 second count.

4. Slowly begin lowering your body to the stretch position, making sure you make the calf muscles endure the negative portion of the resistance.

5. As you reach the bottom position, with the heels pointing to the floor, make sure you do not allow your heels to drop too fast. Go slow and focus on the stretching of the calf muscles.

Standing Calf Raise

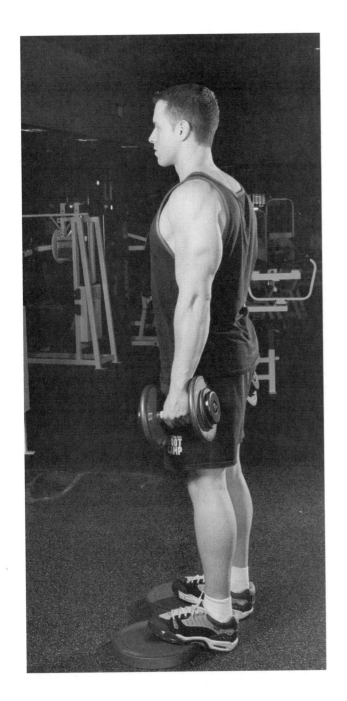
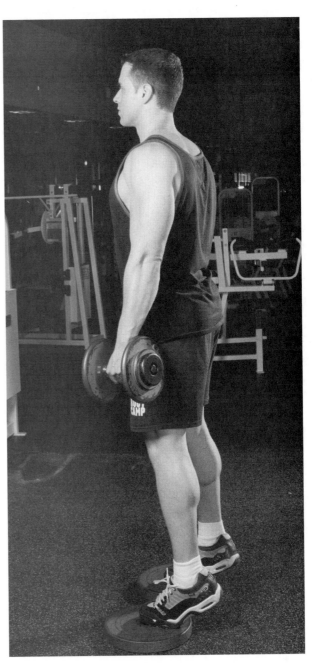

Seated Machine Calf Raise

This exercise primarily targets the soleus muscles underneath the gastrocnemius. This movement is an excellent tool for shaping the calves.

PROPER ALIGNMENT:

1. Choose a weight with which you can practice perfect form. The object is to use good form rather than just trying to lift a gargantuan amount of weight.

2. Sit down and position your feet on the platform.

3. With your feet pointing straight ahead, place your toes and the balls of your feet on the platform.

4. Place the padded support on top of your thighs. Make sure that the pad fits snug against the thigh close to the knee rather than high on top of the thigh.

5. Position your hands on the sides of the thigh pad.

6. Keep your torso straight and do not lean forward or backwards during the exercise.

7. Keep your head straight and level and look straight ahead at all times.

TECHNIQUE AND FORM

1. Once you are in position and ready to begin the exercise, lower your heels toward the floor and slowly bring the calves to a full stretch.

2. Hold this position for a count of 1-2 seconds.

3. From this position, without momentum, push off the balls of your feet and come up on to your tiptoes, pushing as high off the toes as possible. Contract the calves as hard as you possibly can and concentrate all of your efforts on doing so. Hold this position for a 1-2 second count.

4. Slowly begin lowering your body back once again to the stretch position, making sure you make the calf muscles endure the negative portion of the resistance.

5. As you reach the bottom position, with the heels pointing to the floor, make sure you do not allow your heels to drop too fast. Go slow and focus on the stretching of the calf muscles.

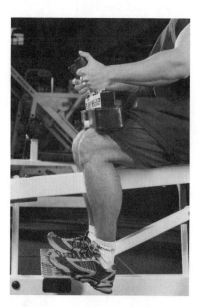

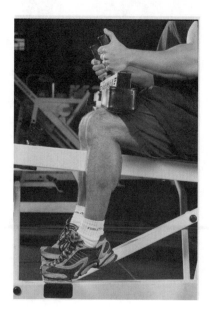

Seated Machine Calf Raise

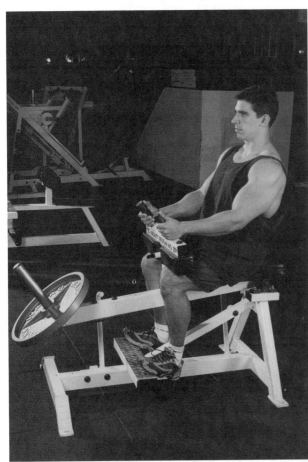

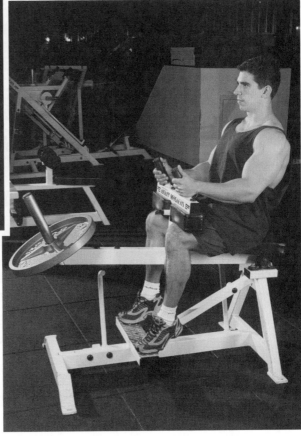

Donkey Calf Raise

This is a great exercise for the calves because it helps to develop the entire calf musculature. You have the option of performing this exercise in a few different ways. One way is with the use of a specially designed machine called the donkey calf press. Another way, which might seem a bit odd, is by using the assistance of another person who actually sits on you!

Most gyms will have a piece of fitness gear called the "Dip Belt". It is a leather belt with an attached chain that allows you to add weight plates. Look at the picture below to see how it looks and how it is used. Instead of using a machine or the assistant, you simply strap the belt to your waist, add weight and begin. Follow the same steps listed below with the exception of #4. To purchase a dip belt, refer to the resource page in the back of the book and visit our web sites for all of your fitness gear needs.

PROPER ALIGNMENT

1. Take a firm grip on a bar or the rail of a staircase.

2. Bend over at the hips, so that your torso is parallel to the floor.

3. Place a 4-5 inch platform or piece of wood beneath your feet.

4. Have your assistant sit upon the lumbar region of your lower back, making sure that it is secure. They must be sure not to move around or one of you could be seriously injured.

TECHNIQUE AND FORM

1. Make sure that you are secure and in stable alignment.

2. Begin by pressing up onto the tips of your toes, focusing on the entire calf area.

3. Press up as high as you can and briefly hold the contraction.

4. Slowly lower yourself, bringing the heels down towards the ground for a deep stretch. Do not go too deep; gauge yourself.

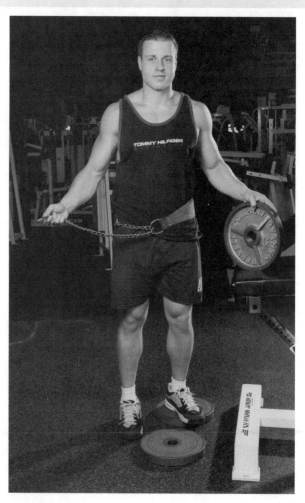

Donkey Calf Raise

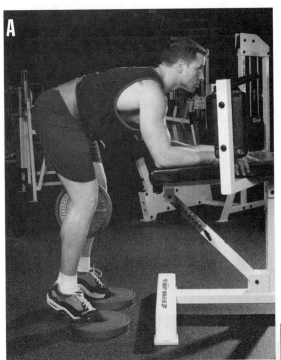

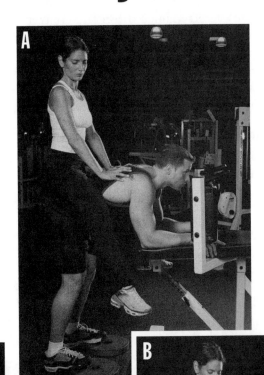

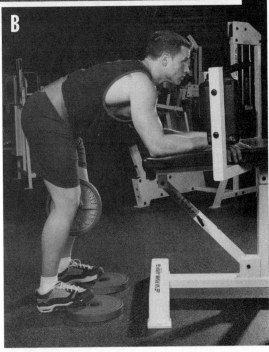

Calf Press

This particular exercise zones in on the gastrocnemius muscles of the calves. It is performed on the same machine where you do your leg presses. This is an excellent alternative to standing calf raises for people that have lower back injuries.

There are two ways to perform this exercise: one leg at a time or both legs at the same time. In this book we will discuss the more common two-legged version. However, the execution for the exercise remains the same for both versions.

PROPER ALIGNMENT

1. Step on to the platform of the machine and place your feet about 3-5 inches apart.

2. Load the machine with the desired resistance.

3. Position your feet on the platform so only the upper edge of your foot rests on the platform. The other half will hang off the platform.

4. Take hold of the handles, usually located to the sides of the machine.

5. Try to keep the legs straight during the exercise with your knees slightly bent.

TECHNIQUE AND FORM

1. Maintaining your form, raise up onto the tips of your toes as high as you can and hold.

2. Focus on contracting the calf muscles at this point. It is one thing to just do the movement, it is another to intensely participate in it!

3. Slowly lower yourself, bringing the heels towards you for a deep stretch. Do not go too deep.

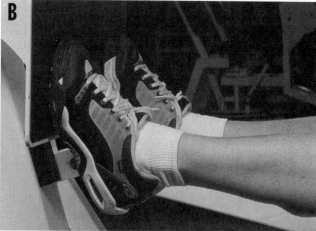

CLOSE UP

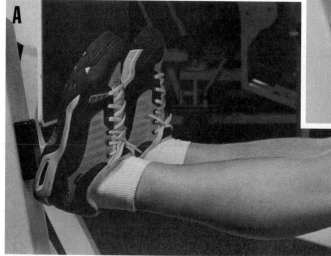

Calf Press

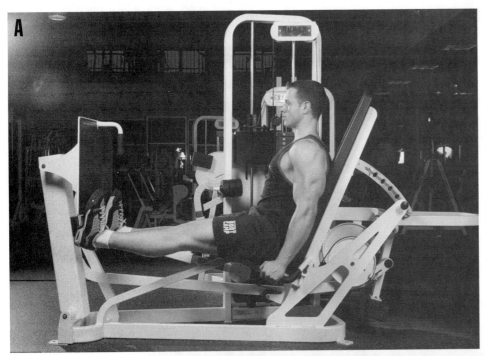

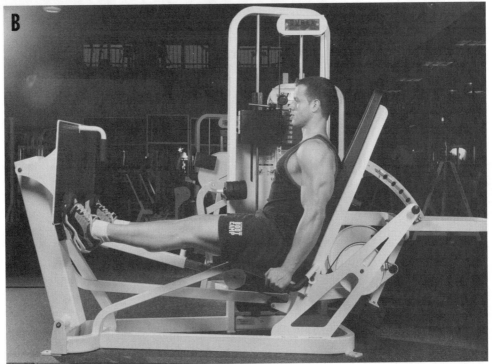

Chapter 7
Back

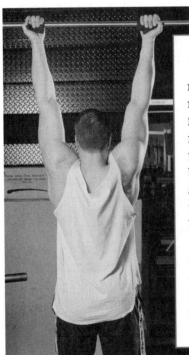

The back is composed of several different muscles. They are the second most neglected muscles by guys (the first being legs) as most figure that what cannot be seen from the front, must not be important. However, we are here to tell you that a well developed back can not only be seen from the front (as lats do get wider) but also creates a powerful V-shaped look that will turn heads. Besides, the wider and thicker your back is, the smaller your waist size looks.

We will focus on the very best exercises for full development of the back region. Pay attention to the proper alignment, technique and form principles as this will help to ensure your success.

7

A WORD ABOUT EXERCISES THAT UTILIZE VARIOUS HAND POSITIONS AND HOW EACH VARIATION CAN AFFECT DIFFERENT MUSCLE GROUPS.

Although many people do not enjoy reading information full of jargon, sometimes we need to learn important facts that in turn will produce the results we wish for. Do not underestimate the power of the information contained below.

Most people do not realize just how powerful a slight variation in your handgrip and hand position on the exercise bar can be. This variation of your hand placement can stimulate completely different areas of muscle concentration.

Whether you choose a wide-grip or narrow-grip, an overhand-grip or an underhand-grip, the area of muscle concentration will in some way be different. The enormous variety of exercise bar attachments available to us further enables us to attach many diversely shaped attachment bars to a pulley cable system. (If you are unaware of the large assortments of attachment bars available to you and how each works, refer to the web site resource page in the back of this book for further information).

You can perform exercise movements that are almost identical to one another, but the difference in exercise bars, hand placement, grip position and the mechanics of the body, will result in stimulating many different muscle groups.

Just as you may not have been able to pull yourself up with the wide-grip pull-up exercise, you might also have difficulty doing a narrow-grip pull-up. If you look at the differences between the wide-grip pull-up and the narrow-grip pull-up, you will notice that the wide-grip pull-up utilizes a wide and overhand grip placement. The narrow-grip pull-up utilizes a narrow and underhand grip placement. Now take a moment and think about what muscles are primarily working when you perform a wide-grip pull-up or a wide-grip pull-down. Because of the overhand-grip you take with these particular exercises, muscles such as the forearm muscles (extensor muscles), shoulder muscles (deltoids), and the back muscles (latissimus dorsi and erector spinae) will take a majority of the work efforts necessary to carryout these movements.

During the underhand narrow-grip pull-up, because of your underhand grip placement, the biceps muscles take the majority role of prime muscles involved during exercise execution. Although your focus should be to keep the biceps from becoming involved too much during this exercise and to instead concentrate on stimulation of the back muscles, it can be extremely difficult, if not impossible to completely avoid the participation of the biceps muscles.

This discussion should begin to help you realize the enormous benefits of practicing the mind/muscle connection and muscle control techniques found within the Zone-Tone method.

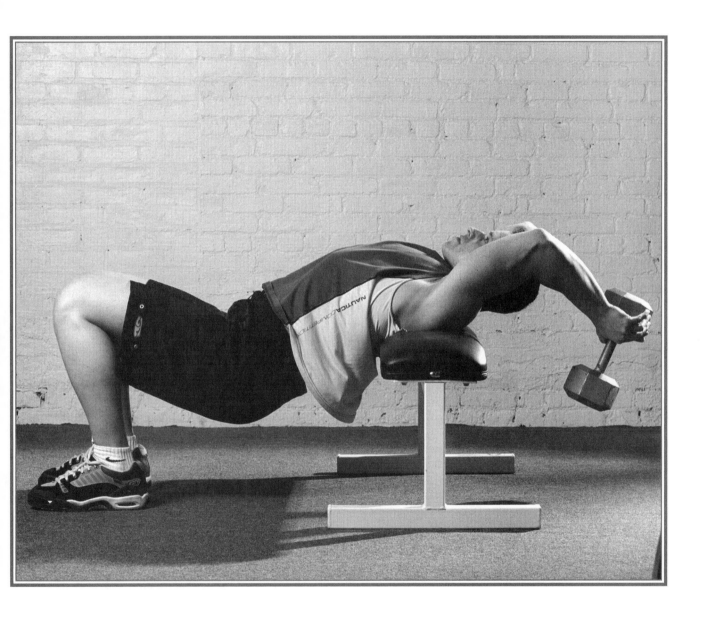

Bent-Over Barbell Row

The bent-over barbell row places primary emphasis on the mid back muscles and the latissimus dorsi with a secondary emphasis on the on the lower back, rear deltoids and biceps. If you follow correct training protocol, you will soon be able to move up in weight. People with lower back problems are better off using the dumbbell version.

PROPER ALIGNMENT

1. Place a bar in front of you on the ground, or on a rack level with your hips. Placing the bar any higher will just make it harder for you to lift it when the weights are increased.

2. Align your feet about shoulder width apart.

3. Make sure your knees are pointing directly in front of you throughout the movement. (Do you notice the similarities in postural and alignment positions for all exercises so far? They are all relatively the same since nothing really changes except for the positions of the body, depending on the exercises performed.)

4. Bend over at the hips, making sure that your lower back is not slumped over. To make sure of this, squeeze or contract your abdominal section while slightly arching your low back, mimicking again yourself sitting in a chair. Do not bend over all the way as this can injure the lower back. Bending at the hips to a position where your upper arm (triceps) can still follow directly towards the ceiling is sufficient for back muscle stimulation. If you stand too upright, this positioning will not sufficiently activate the back muscles. You must be bent over to a degree where the elbows will naturally remain close to the body. At the same time, the back of the arms (triceps) follow a row-like movement, directly towards the ceiling.

5. Pick up the bar using either a palms-down or a palms-up type of grip. The palms-down grip is recommended for beginners as with this grip there tends

to be less biceps involvement. Advanced trainees can benefit from a palms-up grip as it stresses the "lats" in a more direct manner. Also, at the advanced level trainees know how to keep the biceps from getting as involved throughout the performance of the exercise.

6. Stick out your chest while slightly squeezing your shoulder blades together. This will position and keep your body in the proper alignment throughout the movement. Holding these alignment positions throughout the exercise will help make sure that stimulation remains in the back muscles.

7. Keep your head up and looking straight ahead throughout the movement. This will help you keep your balance and make it easier to maintain the described position.

With a few practice sessions, you will be able to perform the exercises with ease. We have noticed once most clients learn to correctly execute exercises they often make dramatic progress within the first few days of beginning the program.

TECHNIQUE AND FORM

As you pick up the bar, think about what muscles you are about to exercise. The latissimus dorsi, also known as the "lats," are located on the outermost side of the back and are a good point focus.

1. Align your body in the correct postural alignment.

2. Let the bar hang down.

3. Keep the elbows slightly wider than shoulder width.

4. Slightly squeeze the shoulder blades together.

5. Begin rowing the elbows up toward the ceiling, allowing the back of the arms (triceps) to lead the motion.

6. Drive the elbows and back of the arms upward until the barbell is touching your lower belly and you are able to fully contract the back muscles. Imagine that there is an egg in the middle of your back. Your objective for each repetition, when the bar is being pulled to your belly, is to crack the egg with your back muscles.

7. Try to squeeze and hold that position for a 2-second count, focusing on an intense contraction of the back muscles. When you consciously squeeze the muscles at the top of the movement, you are simultaneously learning to isolate those specific muscles. When you apply this technique to an exercise, you are actually optimizing your training sessions through the increased muscle recruitment.

8. Begin your descent downward with a slow and controlled movement.

9. As you reach the bottom, slowly and smoothly begin the movement upward again without resting. Make sure that no momentum is involved while changing over from the bottom position to the upward movement. Once again, when your form starts to get sloppy, STOP! Either reduce the weight or take a rest in preparation for the next set.

Bent-Over Barbell Row

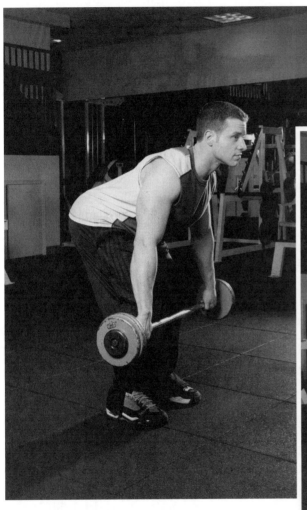

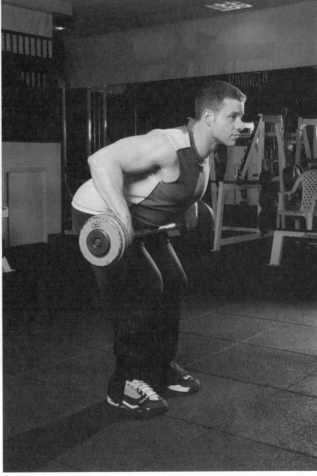

Dumbbell Row

The dumbbell row emphasizes the same set of muscles as the bent over barbell row version with an added benefit of less lower back involvement. In addition, this exercise allows you to focus more on the back muscles because you will be doing one side at a time.

There are two ways to perform this exercise: one arm at a time or both arms at the same time (in which case the exercise will be identical to barbell rows except for the fact that the palms of the hands will be facing your torso). In this book we will discuss the more common one-arm version. This exercise variation is great if you have back problems or are concerned that you have not yet mastered the bent-over row exercise yet.

PROPER ALIGNMENT

This exercise is very similar to the bent-over row. You will be exercising the same muscle group, the back muscle; however, with the dumbbell row your position will be different and you will be exercising one limb at a time as opposed to two.

1. To start, pick up a dumbbell that is light enough to focus primarily on form. Many people find that practicing perfect form with a light weight is much easier than practicing with no weight. The reason for this is because the resistance helps you to feel the desired muscle being exercised, making it easier to isolate and stimulate that muscle. This is another example of the "mind-to-muscle" connection.

2. Find a bench and set the dumbbell at the right side of it.

3. Position your right foot on the floor while positioning your left knee on the bench. Your left hand should be positioned slightly in front of your body on the bench. Lean slightly into your left hand to help support your bodyweight.

Here you will be training the right side of your back.

4. Pick up the dumbbell with your right hand while remembering to support your bodyweight with your left hand.

5. Your back should be parallel to the floor. The back should be flat as you lean over from the hips and you should be looking straight ahead to help maintain balance and form. Do not look down or up during the exercise.

TECHNIQUE AND FORM

As you pick up the dumbbell, think about what muscle you are about to exercise; the right side of the back called the latissimus dorsi, or the "lats."

1. Align your body in the exercise's correct postural alignment.

2. Let the dumbbell hang down.

3. Slightly lift the right shoulder blade, making sure that it maintains a level position.

4. Begin rowing the right elbow up

toward the ceiling, allowing the back of the arms (triceps) to lead the motion.

5. Row the right elbow and back of the right arm up towards the ceiling, and row as far as you can until the back of the arm and elbow reach the level of the torso. Make sure that you are fully contracting the right side of the back muscles. Imagine that there is an egg in the middle of your mid-back. Your objective, when the dumbbell is being rowed, is to squeeze the right side of the back muscles to the left and crack the egg with your back muscles.

6. Try to squeeze and hold that position for a 2-second count, focusing on an intense contraction of the back muscles.

7. Begin your descent with a slow and controlled movement.

8. As you reach the bottom, slowly and smoothly begin the movement upward again without resting. Make sure that no momentum is involved when changing over from the bottom position back to the upward movement. Again, when your form starts to get sloppy, STOP! Either reduce the weight, or take a rest in preparation for the next set.

Dumbbell Row

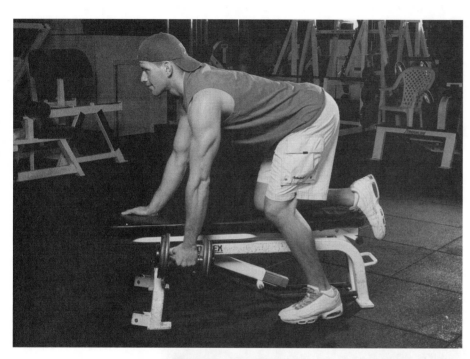

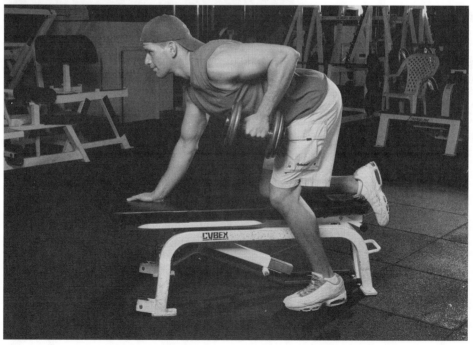

Wide Grip Pull-ups to Front

The pull-up is a very challenging back exercise. However, its ability to deliver quick results and functional upper body strength makes it well worth its weight in gold. Its main emphasis is on the "lats" and the mid-back muscles. There is no involvement of the lower back muscles in this exercise. Secondary muscles involved are the rear deltoids and the biceps.

Note: If you cannot pull your own body weight there are two things that you can do. If your gym has Gravitron machines (machines that assist you in pulling your body weight) feel free to use those. If your health club is not equipped with such machines, then either have someone provide assistance by holding your legs or just use the pull-down machines. Then, when you get strong enough, feel free to start doing pull-ups.

PROPER ALIGNMENT

The pull-up focuses on the natural resistance and mechanics of the body. Too many people perform this exercise incorrectly. They use too much momentum, do not use a full range of motion, or simply do not know the proper technique and form to follow for optimum results.

1. To start, take hold of an overhead bar with an overhand grip.

2. Align your body by spacing your hands about shoulder width apart. It's important to realize that different hand spacing will sometimes focus on one muscle more than another. We recommend a grip 1 1/2 times your shoulder width since it will help keep the biceps from being stimulated and is a great position for back muscle stimulation.

3. Contract your abdominal section, which helps to sustain your postural alignment throughout the movement.

4. Stick your chest out while depressing your shoulders (downward), which will help isolate the intended musculature of the back.

5. Throughout the movement, always keep your head and eyes looking up. Knowing that you must reach your target position at the top adds that extra push.

TECHNIQUE AND FORM

1. Holding onto the bar with an overhand grip 1 1/2 times your shoulder width, let your body hang while bending your knees and crossing your feet.

2. Keep your elbows as wide as you can while you pull your body up.

3. As you are pulling up, make sure your chest is sticking out as much as possible. Your shoulders should be depressed (downward) and as relaxed as possible.

4. When you reach the top (which will be when you can no longer move upward while maintaining the proper alignment), consciously focus on squeezing and contracting the back muscles as hard as you can. Try to hold that contraction for at least 1-1/2 seconds, which will help to isolate the back muscles.

5. As you begin your descent, slowly lower your body while mentally focusing on the back muscles being activated. When you feel yourself fatiguing or losing control on the way down, try to pull back up. You'll notice that as you get tired, even your best attempt to pull yourself back up will not stop your descent. This technique will add some additional intensity and overall stimulation of the back muscles.

6. For a full range of motion, let your arms straighten completely at the bottom of the movement. Most people only come down two-thirds of the way and leave out perhaps the most important portion of the exercise-the fully stretched position. Next, slowly and smoothly begin the transition upward once again without using any momentum.

Wide Grip Pull-ups to Front

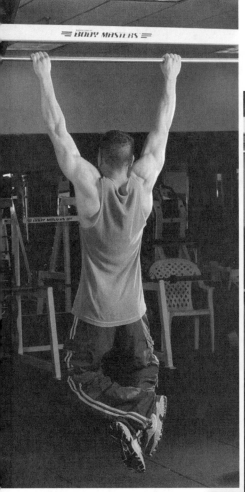

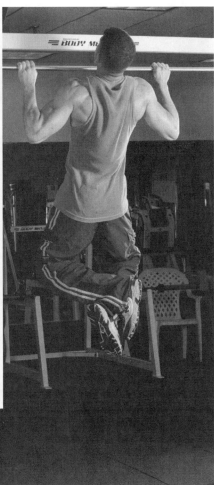

**WIDE GRIP PULL-UP
WITH ASSISTANCE**

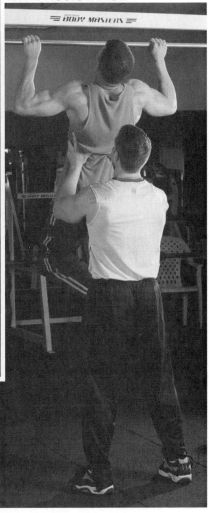

Close-Grip Pull-up

Some people think that similar looking exercises, such as this and the wide-grip pull-up, will affect the same musculature of the back. This couldn't be further from the truth. Wide-grip pull-ups focus on widening the muscles of the upper back and lats. Narrow-grip pull-ups focus more on widening the muscles of the lower lats and also on the serratus muscles (the little finger-like muscles) located on the lower outside of the pecs, near the front of the body.

Avoid making the biceps the primary muscles stimulated in this exercise by focusing on form and concentrating your mind on the back muscles.

PROPER ALIGNMENT

1. Choose your grip of choice, either the parallel close-grip bar or the underhand chin-up. No matter which grip you choose, both of the exercises will be done the same way.

2. Take your grip and focus all of your attention to the lower lat muscles of the back.

3. Hang from the bar with arms at full length. The object of this exercise is to angle your body backwards so that your chest is able to contact the parallel bars or chin-up bar for a greater muscle contraction in the lats.

4. Bend your lower legs at the knees and cross your feet.

5. Stick your chest out as far as possible and lean your head back.

6. The key to isolation of the back muscles and negation of the biceps is to isometrically contract the lat muscles as you hang. The isometric contraction will help activate the lat muscles well before the exercise begins. This will help you to better control and force the lat muscles to become the major muscles being stimulated during the exercise. If you don't know how to isometrically contract the muscles, practice

posing in the mirror without using any weights.

Once you isometrically contract the lats and have set yourself up into the proper alignment, you can begin the exercise.

TECHNIQUE AND FORM

1. First, with your lats already isometrically contracted and your body and head leaning back on an angle, begin slowly pulling your body upwards.

2. As you are driving your way upward to the top of the movement, keep your elbows riding close to your body, rowing them back behind you. You should start to see how the back muscles become stimulated through exercise. The reason you are angled backwards here is so that the elbows can follow their natural arc across and behind the body.

3. At the midway point, moving upward, you should really be feeling the lat muscles working and taking on the majority of your body's resistance. If you don't, stop and practice using light weight on a pull-down machine.

4. As you reach the top of the movement, you should try to touch your

chest on the bar, or at least come close to doing so.

5. Your main objective in this upper position is to contract the lat muscles as hard as you possibly can and hold that position for a count of 1-2 seconds.

6. From this point, it is very important for you to slowly lower yourself from this position. The negative resistance you'll achieve while lowering your body is extremely valuable for overall muscle stimulation. Too many people, simply let their muscles go limp and drop immediately from the top position to the bottom position, completely wasting the valuable negative component of this exercise.

7. As you reach the bottom position, let your arms hang completely straight, allowing for a full and complete stretch of the lats.

8. In this position, without resting, once again isometrically contract the lat muscles. Remember, by activating the lat muscles first, you will help isolate them right from the beginning of the exercise.

9. Align your body and head on an angle leaning backwards and begin pulling upward again in a smooth and fluid motion without using momentum.

Close-Grip Pull-up

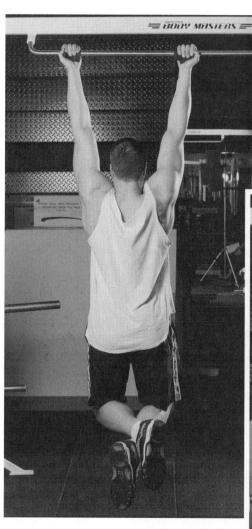

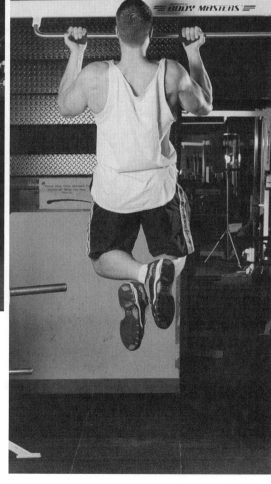

Wide-Grip Pull-Down

If you are not able to pull up your own body weight, you can use the lat pull-down machine to help increase your strength. Although the pull-up is a much better exercise for back muscle development because it works with the body's natural mechanics and range of motion, the pull-down can help prime and get you ready for the pull-up. If you use this exercise, really concentrate on isolating and contracting those back muscles.

PROPER ALIGNMENT

1. Position the thigh support so that you are in a snug position with your feet placed flat on the floor.

2. Choose your desired weight and take a grip equal to twice your shoulder width.

3. Lean back slightly from the hips while contracting the abdominal muscles for support.

4. As you prepare to pull down, stick your chest out while keeping your elbows wide.

5. With a slight lean backwards at the hips, your chest pushed out and your elbows wide, you are ready to begin the exercise.

TECHNIQUE AND FORM

1. Once in position and focused on the muscles of the back, pull the bar down to your collar bone while maintaining your postural alignment.

2. Make sure that you pull the bar down in a smooth, controlled manner, letting

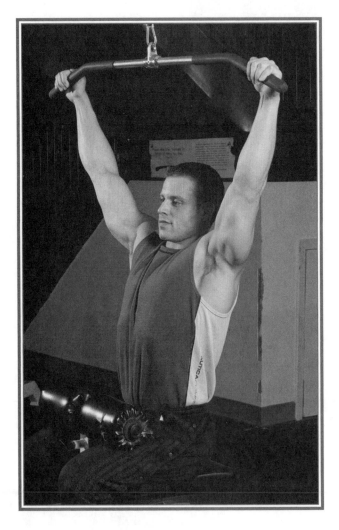

the muscles of the back do the work and not your biceps or momentum. If you don't know the difference between controlled form and momentum already, you will feel the difference in muscle stimulation when you use controlled form.

3. As you reach the bottom of the movement, make sure to squeeze the back muscles for a count of 1 1/2 seconds with the bar close to or touching the collar bone.

4. Slowly begin moving the bar upward and allow it to return to the start position.

5. When you reach the top, do not rest! Immediately begin pulling down making sure you do so slowly while maintaining the correct form and postural alignment. Remember the time under tension principle of continued motion and no rest. You are here to work, not rest. You will accomplish a great deal more by keeping constant tension in the muscle throughout the entire set as opposed to resting at every transition of the top and bottom positions.

Wide-Grip Pull-Down

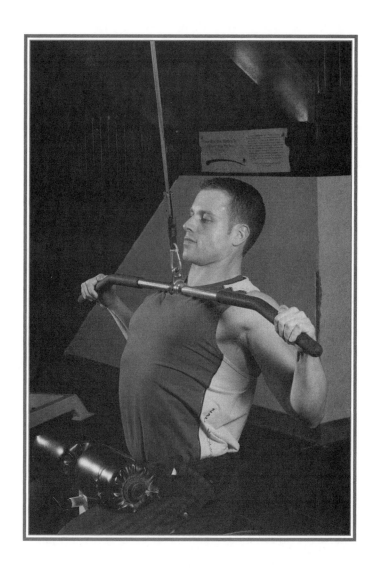

Narrow Grip Pull-Down

During the narrow-grip pull-down exercise, the positioning of your hands will take a different hand position and grip placement when compared to the narrow-grip pull-up. The narrow-grip attachment in the pictures below has two handles that are structured parallel to one another. When you take your hand position, the palms of your hand will be closely facing each other.

As you can clearly see, your whole arm position has now changed in comparison to the narrow underhand-grip pull-up. Notice how close the arms are to one another. You can see how the arms remain close to each other from the beginning of the exercise to the finish position. If you were to perform the narrow-grip exercise and immediately follow with the wide-grip pull-down exercise, you will feel a major difference in the muscles that are stimulated. This is evidence proving how dramatic the variation in bar attachments and your hand placement can be in stimulating different muscles.

The same way you have the option of using the lat pull-down machine to help those men who are not able to do a wide-grip pull-up, the same applies for the men who cannot yet do a narrow-grip underhand pull-up. Here you have the option of performing the narrow-grip pull-down exercise.

PROPER ALIGNMENT

1. Position the thigh support so that you are in a snug position with your feet placed flat on the floor.

2. Choose your desired weight and take your desired narrow grip that we discussed above.

3. Lean back slightly from the hips while slightly contracting the abdominal muscles for support.

4. As you prepare to pull down, stick your chest out while keeping your elbows narrow and close to your body.

5. With a slight lean backwards at the hips, your chest pushed out and your elbows staying close to your body, you are ready to begin the exercise.

TECHNIQUE AND FORM

1. Once in position and focused on the muscles of the back, pull the bar down to your upper chest region, while maintaining your postural alignment.

2. Make sure that you pull the bar down in a smooth, controlled manner, letting the muscles of the back do the work, while trying to avoid your biceps or momentum from becoming involved. If you don't know the difference between controlled form and momentum already, you will surely feel the difference in muscle stimulation when you use correct controlled form.

3. As you reach the bottom of the movement, make sure to squeeze the back muscles for a count of 1 1/2 seconds with the bar close to or touching the upper chest region.

4. Slowly begin allowing the bar to move in its upward descent, returning back to the start position.

5. When you reach the top, do not rest! Immediately begin pulling back down, making sure you do so slowly while maintaining the correct form and postural alignment. Remember the time under tension principle of continued motion and no rest. You are here to work, not rest. You will accomplish a great deal more by keeping constant tension on the muscles, throughout the entire set as opposed to resting at every transition of the top and bottom positions.

Narrow Grip Pull-Down

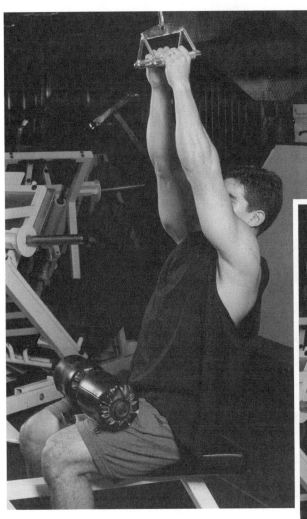

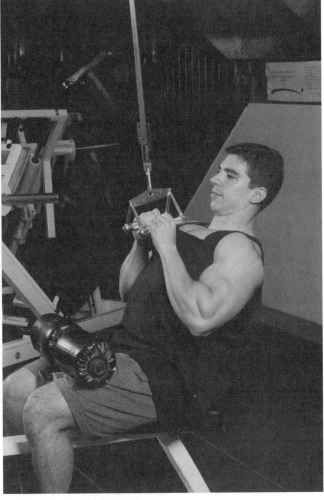

Seated Low-Pulley Row

(Lower Lats and Mid-Back Muscles)
Using a close-grip parallel attachment

The low-pulley row is an exercise that most people perform incorrectly. They either lean too far forward in the beginning or too far backwards at the top, taking the stress off the lat muscles, or they use momentum instead of muscle to move the weight. You can choose a variety of different handles for this exercise. Each one hits a slightly different area of the back, providing a great variety for an exciting and never stale back routine. The description of technique and form below assumes that you will be using a close-grip parallel bar attachment.

PROPER ALIGNMENT

1. Once you attach the bar to the pulley system, take a seat on the machine bench.

2. Choose a weight that will allow you to practice perfect form while also providing enough weight to stimulate the back muscles. Using too light a weight will keep you from feeling the desired muscle stimulation.

3. Take hold of the bar, either leaning forward or having someone hand it to you.

4. Sit straight up while you bend at the knees.

5. Plant your feet evenly on each side of the platform and point them straight ahead.

6. Slightly contract the abdominal muscles.

7. Stick your chest out and retract the scapula and shoulder blades.

8. Keep your elbows close to your body and hands down by your lower abdominals.

9. Keep your head level and look straight ahead throughout the movement.

TECHNIQUE AND FORM

1. First, to avoid lower-back injury, make sure that your knees are bent and that you don't lean too far forward. A very slight lean forward is okay.

2. With the arms fully stretched forward, retract the scapula from this position. This will pre-isolate the lat muscles of the back.

3. Your objective will be to pull the bar back to your lower-to-mid abdominal section, making sure you adhere to the following steps.

4. You will want to keep the elbows riding close to the body, helping to stimulate the back muscles. The farther you bring the arms away from the body, the less the desired muscles will be stimulated.

5. As you begin pulling the bar toward your abdominal section, stick your chest out as far as it will go while you strive to sit straight up. Do not lean backwards.

6. Concentrate completely on the lat muscles of the back so they do most of the work.

7. When the bar reaches your abdominal section squeeze the back muscles as hard as you possibly can. Picture having an egg planted square in the middle of your back. While the bar is touching your abdominal section, your main objective, while contracting the muscles of the back as hard as you can, will be to squeeze your shoulder blades together so hard that the egg breaks.

8. Hold the contracted position for a count of two seconds.

9. From the contracted position, slowly begin your return to the starting position with a slow and controlled movement.

10. As you reach the starting position, slowly and smoothly begin pulling the bar towards you without resting. Maintain the same form as when you began the exercise, making sure that no momentum is involved while changing over from the contracted position to the starting position.

Seated Low-Pulley Row

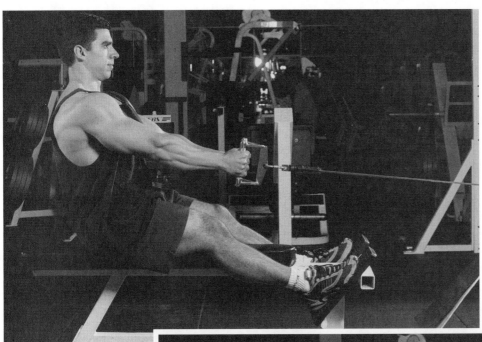

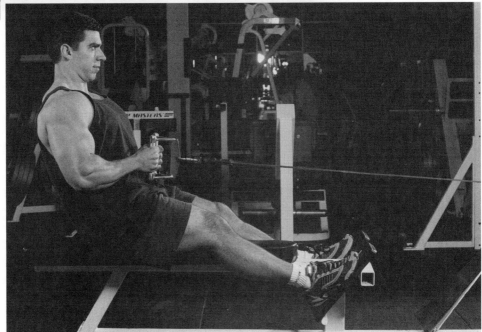

Dumbbell Pullover

Although this exercise looks a little strange, it's great for the upper body. There are two variations: one that focuses mostly on the chest muscles and one that focuses mostly on the back muscles. In this section, we will be discussing the variation that focuses on the back. Please pay attention to the exercise description steps below to help differentiate between the two exercise variations. Not only will this exercise help to create a powerful and thick looking back region, but it will also benefit the triceps muscles located in the back of your arms.

PROPER ALIGNMENT

1. Lie with your body across a flat bench.

2. Ensure that your neck and your upper back are the only body parts resting on the bench.

3. Lift a dumbbell overhead and hold it at arm's length right in front of your face. (Please ensure that the dumbbells you are using have their weights properly secured).

TECHNIQUE AND FORM

1. Slowly lower the dumbbell over your head in an arc.

2. Ensure that your hips are not being raised as you lower the weight.

3. When you reach the fully stretched position, hold the stretch for a second and start raising the weight back up in an arc until you reach the starting position once again.

CHEST

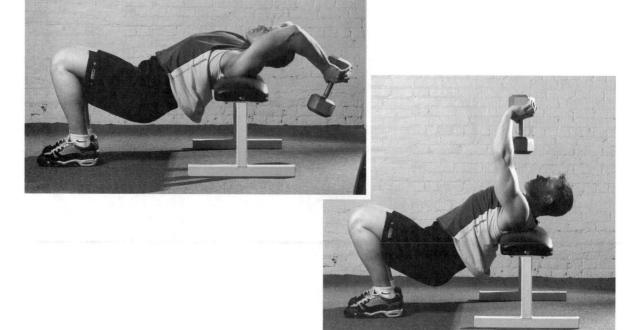

Dumbbell Pullover

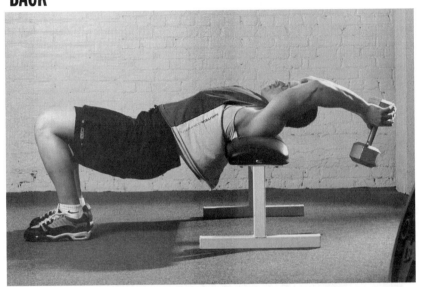

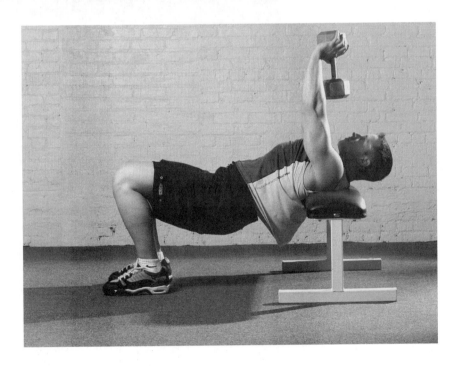

Straight Arm Pull-Down

This is a great isolation exercise for the back as it allows you to work it without the involvement of secondary muscles such as the biceps. In addition, you get the added bonus of working the abs indirectly as you will need to contract them in order to maintain the position required to perform the exercise.

PROPER ALIGNMENT

1. Stand in front of a pull-down bar with your arms extended in front of you holding on to the bar at shoulder width using a palms down grip.

2. In order to gain stability, bend your legs slightly at the knees, contract your abdominals and keep your weight at the heels.

3. Keep the elbows slightly bent and the wrists in a locked position.

4. Maintain a comfortable and forward tilt of the upper body in order to maintain stability throughout the movement.

TECHNIQUE AND FORM

1. Push the bar down toward the body in an arc, making sure that you are only moving from the shoulder joint and not extending at the elbow. There must be no movement at the elbow joint. It must be locked securely in place.

2. Contract your lats as you lower the bar towards your thighs.

3. As soon as the bar touches your thighs, hold the position for a second or two and then slowly go back to the starting position.

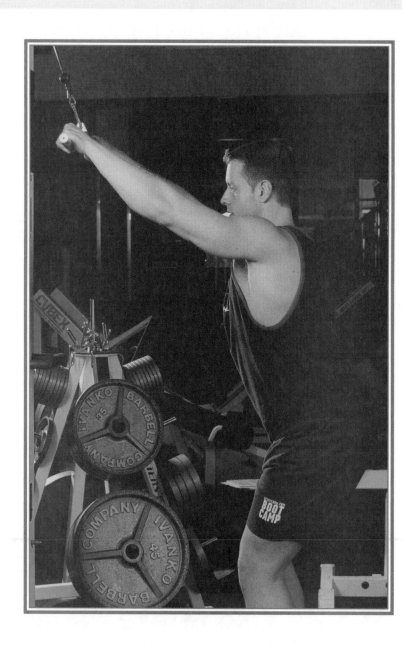

Straight Arm Pull-Down

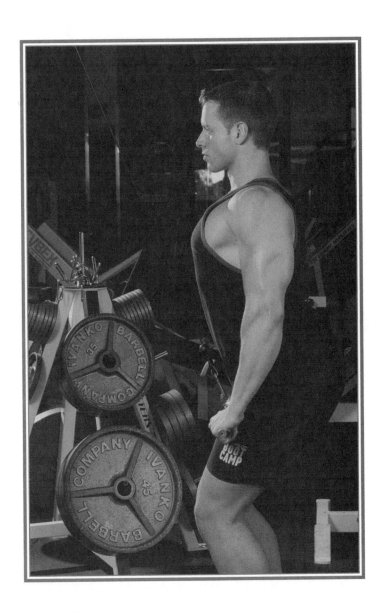

Chapter 8
Chest

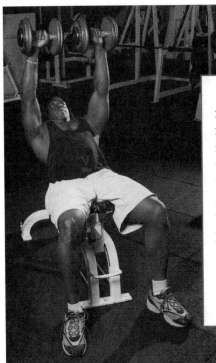

There are many misconceptions when it comes to men and chest training. While most guys think that the flat bench press is the exercise that will provide them with the big chest they are looking for, it is the incline bench press that will deliver the goods. The reason for that is because when you develop a large upper chest, you create the optical illusion of having a gigantic looking chest. If you don't believe me then just look at pictures of Arnold Schwarzenegger and Lee Haney. You will notice that both have huge upper pecs.

8

THE BODY SCULPTING BIBLE FOR MEN

There are four areas of the chest that men should be emphasizing the most:

a) Upper Chest Area with exercises such as the Incline Dumbbell Press.

b) Overall Pec Area with exercises such as the dumbbell press, chest dips and push-ups.

c) Outer Chest Upper Area with exercises such as the Incline Dumbbell Flyes.

d) Inner Upper Chest Area with exercises such as the Incline Cable Crossovers.

We will mostly recommend dumbbells for the performance of chest exercises for several reasons:

They allow for both a greater range of motion and a deeper stretch at the bottom of the movements.

They allow for better isolation and muscle contraction at the top of the movements, helping to recruit more muscle fibers within the chest and surrounding musculature.

They are harder to control and hold than a barbell, helping to strengthen and develop the extremely important antagonistic and synergistic muscles of the chest and shoulders. Overall, the benefits you'll receive from using dumbbells outweigh the barbell by a long shot.

PROPER ALIGNMENT

The postural alignment is basically the same for all of the following chest exercises. However, you will notice differences in some of the following positions, techniques and forms. The most important thing to remember is to always consciously focus and contract the muscles of the chest while maintaining the postural alignment and form during all of the exercises. This will help to stimulate the chest muscles during exercise.

The following sequence of movements will ensure that you learn how to properly lift a dumbbell off the ground and into position to start many of the exercises we describe. It will also demonstrate how to bring the dumbbells back to the start position of an exercise when you have completed it from a lying position. This is an invaluable technique to learn and can prevent many injuries from occurring.

1. When you pick up dumbbells, make sure to bend at the knees while you lift the weight with your legs.

2. Lift with your legs, not with your back! You can easily injure your lower back by bending over to pick up the weight.

3. While standing, place the bottom plate of the dumbbells against your thighs and keep them there as you sit on the bench seat. You will find that by keeping the dumbbells against your thighs as you sit, it will allow you to easily manipulate them to the top of your thighs.

4. Begin positioning your body into the correct postural alignment, starting from the bottom of your body and moving to the top.

5. Space your feet about shoulder width apart.

6. Make sure your knees are pointing straight ahead throughout the movement.

7. As you raise the dumbbells to the starting position on top of your thighs, do not try to muscle them up with your arm muscles. This will only drain your strength and can easily cause an injury. You need 100 percent of your strength for the exercise itself and cannot afford to waste it on something that you can easily avoid. To properly raise the dumbbells from

your thighs into exercise position, follow these guidelines; you will be using
your leg muscles and momentum to
help place you and the dumbbells into
position. While sitting in an upright
position, with the dumbbells on your
thighs, thrust one leg up, leveraging
one dumbbell up to around your
chest level.

8. Immediately thrust the second dumbbell upward, while simultaneously
allowing momentum and the dumbbells to guide you back into the lying
position while your abdominal muscles help safely ease you into that
position. The reason for lying back
immediately when the second dumbbell is thrust upward is so you do not
injure your shoulder joints or lower
back from having to hold the dumbbells in that otherwise awkward position. Lying back immediately following
the dumbbell's momentum while
allowing the abdominal muscles to
ease you into position will help ensure
your safety and keep your strength at
its peak for the exercise. This may
sound difficult, but it's not. It is the
safest and easiest way of getting the
dumbbells into position (especially if
you're using heavy dumbbells).

9. Once you've gotten the dumbbells up,
lay back, until your back touches the
bench.

10. The dumbbells should now be in position at the sides of your chest.

11. Again make sure your feet are shoulder width apart, and that they are flat
on the ground at all times.

12. Make sure your knees are straight.

13. Your lower back should be flat against
the bench at all times, with no excessive arch in the lower lumbar region
(small of the back).

14. Make sure your back is flat against the
bench, with the arms and elbows out to
the sides and the forearms perpendicular to the floor. When you're correctly
positioned, retract or squeeze the shoulder blades together. At first it may seem
uncomfortable or odd, but do not underestimate the significance of this technique. You must learn to hold this position throughout the movement, and
consistent practice will ensure this. By
squeezing the shoulder blades together
and keeping your entire back in constant contact with the bench, you will
actually be taking the anterior shoulder
out of the exercise. The chest muscles
will now be the primary muscles lifting
the weight.

15. Relax your head throughout the movement, and make sure you do not twist it
or lift it from the bench while engaged in
the exercise. Alignment is generally the
same for all of the exercises.

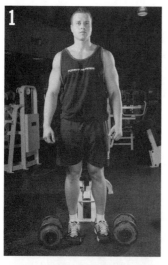

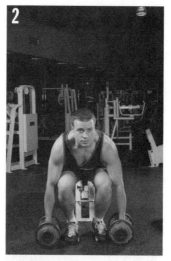

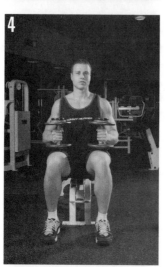

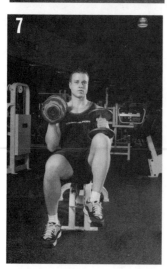

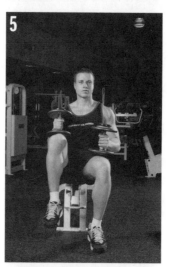

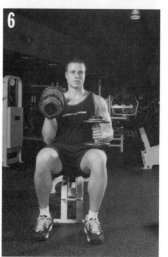

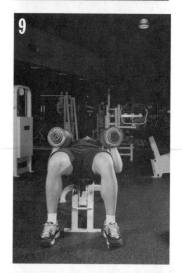

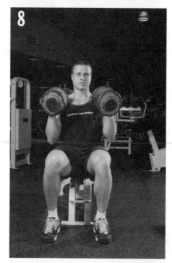

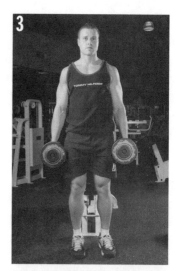

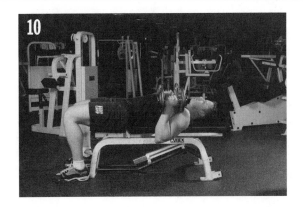

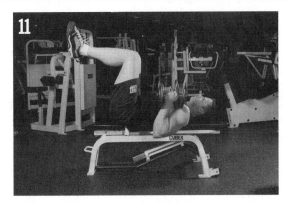

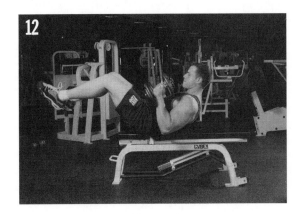

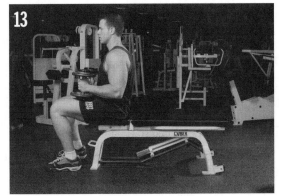

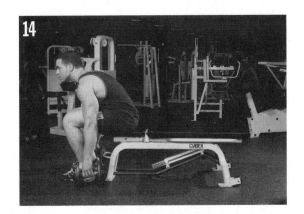

Incline Dumbbell Press

This is an excellent exercise for the upper pectoral muscles. The dumbbells are more challenging than the barbells as they involve stabilizer muscles needed in order to keep the weights in balance. The exercise can be performed in two manners for variety: with palms facing away or palms facing each other. For both variations, the only difference is the position of the palms throughout the movement. However, the movement itself remains the same.

You will notice how you have the option of either touching the dumbbells at the top of the movement or keeping them separated when you reach the top of the movement. This is mostly preference and you will discover yours soon. Some people feel the ability to get a better muscular contraction in the chest muscles when they touch them at the top, while others feel like it is a waste of valuable time and strength. Try both and see what works better for you.

TECHNIQUE AND FORM

1. With the dumbbells on your thighs, thrust one leg up, leveraging one dumbbell up to about your chest level.

2. Immediately thrust the second dumbbell upward while simultaneously allowing momentum and the dumbbells to guide you back into the angled, incline position. Use your abdominal muscles to help safely ease you into that position.

3. As you are lying on the inclined bench, align your body as you were instructed above.

4. Position the dumbbells out to the side of your chest, keeping your elbows wide and your forearms perpendicular to the floor throughout the exercise movement. Find a position that is wide enough to be comfortable and not so wide as to redirect the force to the shoulders. Some trainers believe that bringing the arms out excessively to the sides of the body will help to better isolate the chest muscles. This is a misconception that can actually inhibit chest development and worse, cause injury. The wider you go beyond a comfortable position, the more likely you are to redirect the force of the weight on to the shoulders rather than the pecs. Even worse, when you widen your arms excessively and then proceed to press a heavy or even moderate weight,

you are actually causing the outer pectoral muscle to tear. Once again, bring your arms out to the side of your body to a point where they are still positioned wide, but not excessively!

5. Because the incline dumbbell press positions you on an inclined angle, your shoulder muscles are more likely to move the weight rather than the chest muscles. To avoid this, not only will you want to retract the shoulder blades back or together against the bench; but you must also depress or press the shoulders downward. This slight variation will take the shoulders out of the chest movement, allowing the chest to be the primary area worked during the exercise.

6. With the chest in its elevated position, the elbows out and wide and the forearms perpendicular to the floor, press the dumbbells up toward the ceiling.

7. As you reach the top of the exercise, you can either touch the dumbbells together or press them straight up like a bench press. You can play around with different positions at the top of the movement as you may get a better muscle contraction varying the dumbbell positions. Two people may use two different dumbbell variations in order to fully stimulate their chest muscles. The most important thing you are con-

cerned with is getting the most intense contraction possible! There are a couple of different ways to do this. You can simply touch the dumbbells together and squeeze, or you can turn the dumbbells slightly inward at the top of the movement, allowing for a controlled and isolated contraction. Are you starting to see how you can apply the many new tools of this program to any and all facets of your training regimen?

8. Begin lowering the weight while holding your proper postural alignment throughout the exercise.

9. As your elbows and the back of your arms are lowered, bring the dumbbells to a level that is comfortable, making sure that the chest muscles hold the majority of the resistance. If you don't have any type of shoulder injuries or muscle impingement, you may allow the dumbbells to lower to a comfortable stretch where the dumbbells are parallel with your chest. Always make sure that you stay in control of the dumbbells and maintain this control throughout the exercise.

10. Once you reach the bottom position, slowly begin to press the dumbbells up again in a controlled, smooth and fluid motion without using any momentum.

Incline Dumbbell Press

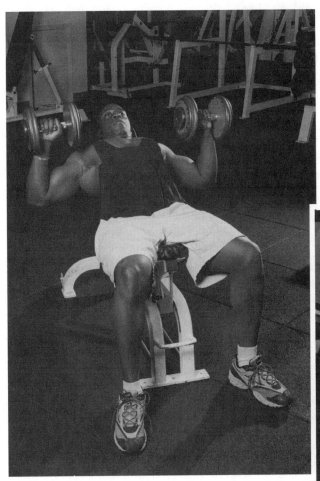

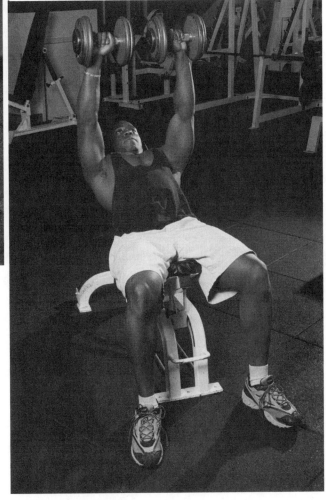

Flat Dumbbell Press

This exercise primarily targets the muscles of the middle chest. As you will soon discover, the fact that you may be able to hoist very heavy weights with the barbell bench press does not necessarily mean that you will be able to do the same over here. At the end of this exercise, it is crucial that you use the techniques we present on how to handle the dumbbells as we have met many people that injure their shoulders from using incorrect techniques at the time of getting the dumbbells back to their starting position.

TECHNIQUE AND FORM

This exercise requires you to use the same technique as the incline dumbbell press, but there will be some slight variations in your postural alignment. You will align your body the same way you did before, but now you will obviously be in a flat position. You'll want to focus more on retracting the shoulder blades rather than depressing them. Otherwise, follow the same technique and form for this exercise as you learned for the incline press.

1. With the dumbbells on your thighs, thrust one leg up, leveraging one dumbbell up to about your chest level. Immediately thrust the second dumbbell upward while simultaneously allowing momentum and the dumbbells to guide you back into the lying, supine position (flat, with your body facing the ceiling). Use your abdominal muscles to safely ease you into that position.

2. Lay back and align your body as you were instructed above.

3. Position the dumbbells to the outside of your chest, keeping the elbows wide and the forearms perpendicular to the floor throughout the exercise movement.

4. Because your shoulder muscles are more likely to move the weight than your chest muscles, you must retract the shoulder blades back or together against the flat bench. This slight variation will take the shoulders out of the chest movement, allowing the chest to be the primary area working during the exercise.

5. With the chest in its elevated position, the elbows out and wide and the forearms perpendicular to the floor, press the dumbbells up toward the ceiling.

6. As you reach the top of the exercise, you can either touch the dumbbells together (as shown on image B) or press them straight up (as shown on

image C) like a bench press. You can play around with different positions at the top of the movement as you may get a better muscle contraction varying the dumbbell positions. Two people may use two different dumbbell variations in order to fully stimulate their chest muscles. The most important thing you are concerned with is getting the most intense contraction possible! There are a couple of different ways to do this. You can simply touch the dumbbells together and squeeze, or you can turn the dumbbells slightly inward at the top of the movement, allowing for a more controlled and isolated contraction.

7. Begin lowering the weight while holding your proper postural alignment throughout the exercise.

8. As your elbows and the back of your arms reach parallel or bench level, slowly begin to press the dumbbells up again in a controlled, smooth, fluid motion, without using any momentum.

Flat Dumbbell Press

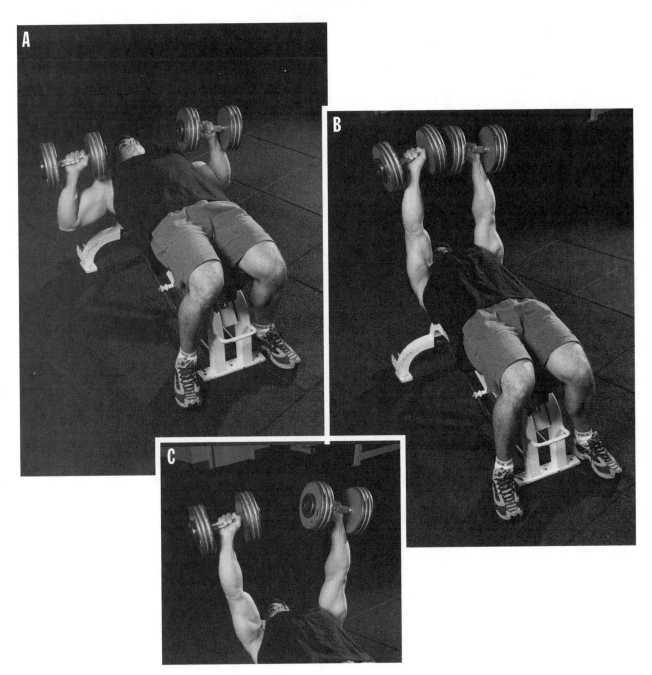

Flat Dumbbell Fly

This exercise is truly a great one. It might seem a bit hard to master, but once you do, it will be a pleasure to perform. It might look as if this exercise is identical to the dumbbell bench press, but it is not. With the dumbbell press, you are extending at the elbow joint and utilizing something called horizontal adduction—a movement together—of the shoulder joints. The dumbbell fly must only incorporate the shoulder joints movement and not the elbow joints extension. The elbows must be locked into place to allow the true magic to begin. The flat dumbbell fly focuses on the mid-chest muscles.

TECHNIQUE AND FORM

For this exercise, your postural alignment will be very similar to the other two chest exercises. However, this exercise will require you to use a different technique and form. With this exercise you will retract the shoulder blades just as you did in the flat and incline dumbbell press, but the angle of the movement is changed. Instead of using the combination of horizontal shoulder adduction (when the shoulders move inward), and elbow extension (when the elbows themselves flex and extend during pressing) as you would in the pressing movements above, for this exercise you'll lock the elbow joint in place. You will set up the arms just as you would for the flat dumbbell press with the arms wide and forearms perpendicular to the floor, but having the elbow locked will prevent any elbow extension or flexion. This technique will exclude the triceps from being involved in the exercise while focusing the resistance completely within the chest muscles.

1. You'll want to align your body exactly as you did with the flat dumbbell press, but now you will have the palms of your hands facing each other instead of facing the wall in front of you.

2. This time you'll be using a visualization technique while engaged in the movement of the exercise. As you begin to squeeze the dumbbells towards each other, you will be following an arch-shaped movement. As you follow this arch, I want you to picture yourself hugging a tree. In other words, make believe there is a tree between you and the dumbbells; you will be mimicking the exact motion of hugging it. This visualization technique will help keep you in the correct position to follow the arch movement. All of this will ensure that your chest muscles receive the most intense stimulation and contraction possible.

3. As you reach the top of the movement, be sure to consciously contract the chest muscles as hard as you possibly can for maximum muscle stimulation!

4. Begin lowering the weight while holding the proper alignment, technique and form throughout the movement. As you reach the bottom of the movement, be sure not to let the back of the arms go too far below the level of the flat bench as this could cause injury to the shoulders' rotator cuff. When you do reach the bottom of the movement, slowly begin squeezing the dumbbells upward in an arch again with a smooth, controlled, fluid motion, making sure that you avoid using momentum!

Flat Dumbbell Fly

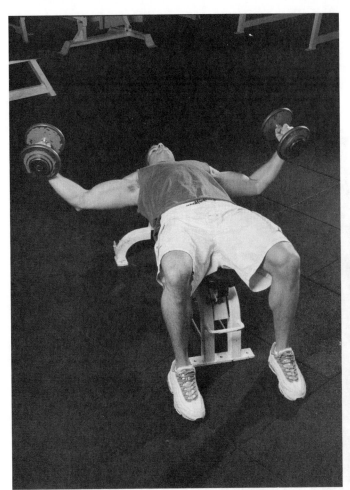

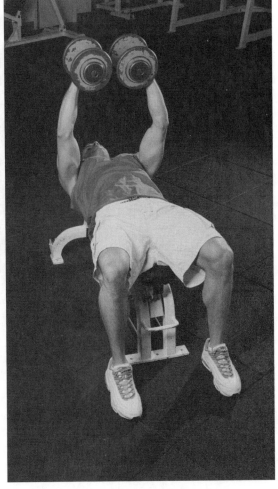

Incline Dumbbell Fly

This exercise is virtually identical to the flat dumbbell fly with the exception that it will focus on the upper chest muscles. Remember that no matter what anyone tells you, it is impossible to avoid hitting muscles located in the same muscle groups. For example, if you are focusing on you lower abdominal muscles, you will inevitably be stimulating the upper abdominal muscles as well. It is great to zone in on the exact muscles you desire to train, but don't be surprised when other parts of the same muscle group are also feeling the work.

TECHNIQUE AND FORM

Follow the same technique and form as for the Flat Dumbbell Flys but use the Incline Bench instead of the Flat Bench. In addition, as a way to increase stimulation of the upper chest, don't let your palms face each other. In other words, your initial position will be the same as the one used for the Incline Dumbbell Press. However, the movement will be the same as the one used for the Flat Dumbbell Fly.

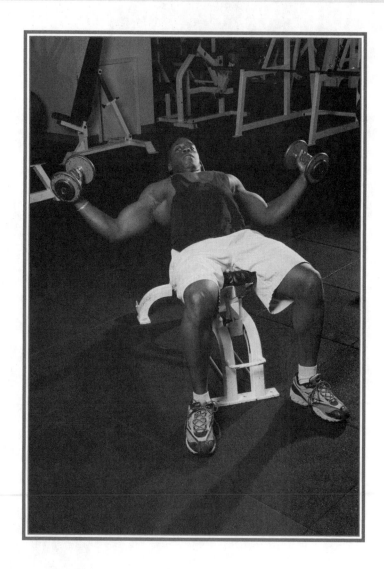

Incline Dumbbell Fly

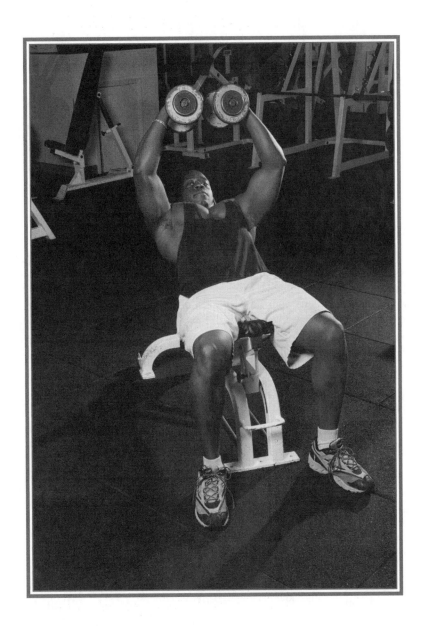

Chest Dip

(Using a parallel dip station)

The chest dip is a great muscle-enhancing exercise that focuses on the lower chest and serratus muscles. Between dips and close grip chins you hit all upper body muscles! There is a major difference between the triceps dip and the chest dip. When we discuss the triceps dips later, we tell you to keep your entire body in a pin straight line, which helps to focus the majority of resistance on your triceps muscles. With the chest dips, we are only concerned with affecting the muscles of the chest. If you cannot do a dip, you might want to try using a weight assistant machine such as the Gravitron, which counter balances a portion of your body weight.

PROPER ALIGNMENT

With this exercise, you'll want to bend at the knees, lock your feet and bend forward as you lower yourself. You must stay bent over to keep the focus of resistance in the chest muscles. These three steps will help transfer most of the resistance to the chest muscles and avoid triceps muscle recruitment. To do this, you will need a dip station or machine. If you are working out in your home, I suggest you purchase an inexpensive dip unit from one of the sports-related retail chains or a wholesale fitness supply store. In a wholesale store, you can usually negotiate a lower price and the quality of the apparatus is usually much better. Look in your local yellow pages for the store nearest you.

1. Place your hands on the parallel bars as you position yourself for postural alignment.

2. The best way to align yourself is to raise yourself up onto the dip bars by locking out your arms. You will then align your body, starting with your head and moving down to your feet.

3. While suspended in the top position of the exercise, your head will at first be level and looking straight ahead. You may find that bending your head slightly forward as you lower yourself will help you lean forward for increased muscle stimulation in the chest. You must constantly focus all of your atten-

tion on the chest muscles during this exercise as this will help increase the involvement of the chest muscles and keep you in the proper alignment.

4. Bend your legs at the knees and hook your feet over one another. This will help keep your back arched forward for the ultimate involvement of the chest muscles. Your arms and elbows will ride away from your body as you lower yourself and when pushing upward to the lockout position. This will help keep the triceps muscles from becoming involved with the exercise.

TECHNIQUE AND FORM

1. Make sure that you have correct postural alignment. Begin the exercise once you are in position with your arms locked out (only in the beginning and end) and your body suspended from the floor.

2. As you lower yourself from the lockout position immediately begin to lean forward. The farther you lean forward, the more your chest muscles will work.

3. Lower yourself slowly while resisting your bodyweight all the way to the bottom position.

4. Keep the elbows and arms away from your body, helping to better isolate the chest muscles and avoid recruiting the triceps muscles.

5. Lower yourself until the backs of your arms are parallel or slightly beyond parallel with the floor.

Remember, you should never go so low that you feel any chest or shoulder pain or you could seriously injure yourself. Go to a point where you are comfortable and increase a little more the next session if needed.

6. When you reach the bottom position, do not rest! Slowly, with a smooth transition, begin to press your body upward without using any momentum. Make sure that you maintain your postural alignment.

7. As you begin pressing upward, make sure that all of your focus is once again directed to your chest muscles. This alone will help stimulate the triceps through increased muscle control. As you near the top of the motion, your goal is not to lock out the joint but to contract and squeeze the chest muscles as hard as you possibly can for a 1 second count. It is important for the chest muscles to hold you in this position rather than lock out with the triceps or the elbow joints.

8. Remember that there should be no rest at the top of the exercise after the contraction period. From that lock out position, once again slowly lower yourself as you resist the weight of your body back to the bottom position. If you get to a point where your body weight is too light for the exercise, you may use a dip belt to hook some additional weight to your body, thus increasing the resistance. Please make sure that if you do use additional weight, you do so in small incremental stages.

Chest Dip

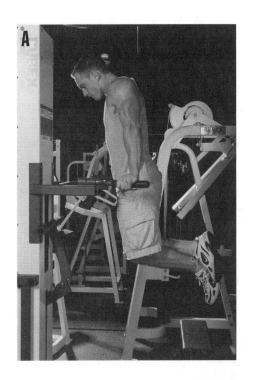

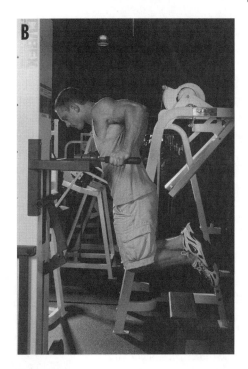

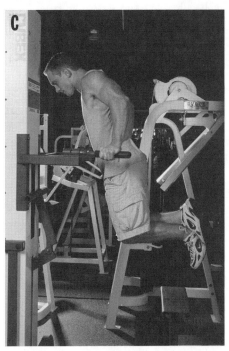

Incline Cable Crossover

Incline cable crossovers are very similar to the dumbbell fly, but there is a major advantage when you perform the incline cable crossover exercise. Only in the beginning of the dumbbell fly exercise is the majority of the resistance placed upon the chest muscles. This soon changes when the dumbbells are brought vertical (arms and dumbbells extended over the chest). At this point, instead of the pecs being responsible for sustaining the resistance of the dumbbells, the elbow joints and shoulders are. The force of gravity disappears when the arms are brought to this vertical position. Cable crossovers don't have this disadvantage. In fact, the degree of resistance remains constant throughout the entire movement.

Performing incline cable crossovers provides even greater benefits than the results obtained from doing regular cable crossovers. Incline cable crossovers add to the development of the upper chest muscles, and give you the appearance of a much larger chest overall. This exercise develops the pectoralis major and minor.

PROPER ALIGNMENT

1. Set the pin to the desired resistance and attach the handles to the cables.

2. If possible, set the pulley level to a height just below your upper chest. This will allow for a more focused contraction in the upper pecs. If you are not able to adjust the pulley height, this is fine, but make sure to keep the focus on the upper pecs.

3. Take hold of the handles with an overhand grip and position yourself so that you are in the middle of the pulley machine (in order to position yourself in the middle of the machine, you must pull each of the handles closer to you, thus lifting both weight stacks simultaneously.)

4. Make sure that both weight stacks are even on the right and left sides. Do not allow the weight stacks to become uneven or you will create a muscle imbalance when you begin the exercise.

5. With the handles in hand, palms facing each other and standing in the middle of the machine, bend your elbows slightly and lock them there throughout the exercise.

6. You will begin this exercise in the extended position (arms opened up as if about to give a hug) as opposed to the dumbbell fly where you started in a flexed (contracted) position.

7. Keep a slight bend in the knees to prevent lower-back strain.

8. Remember, you must maintain this perfect alignment so select a weight light enough to maintain form throughout the movement.

TECHNIQUE AND FORM

1. You should be positioned in the middle of the cable crossover and parallel to the weight stacks with the hand grips in hand and arms extended out to the sides of your body. The resistance will provide a nice stretch to the pec muscles.

2. To begin the exercise, keep the arms slightly bent and contract the chest muscles.

3. Bring the cables across and in front of the body until the two handgrips touch at the level of or just above your upper chest.

4. Make sure to contract the chest muscles as hard as possible in this position and hold for a one second count.

5. Once the two hands touch and you have forcefully contracted the chest muscles, let the resistance of the weight stacks bring the arms back to the starting position in a slow controlled manner.

6. Repeat the movement.

Incline Cable Crossover

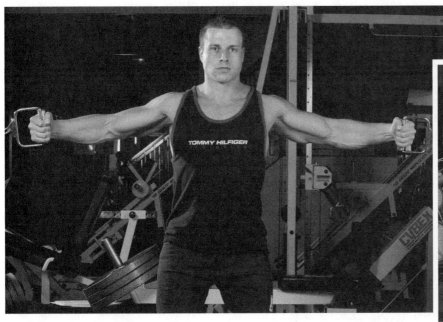

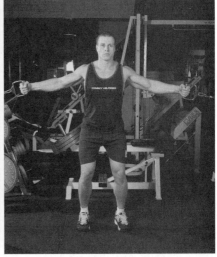

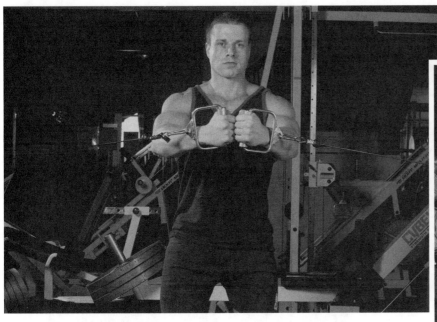

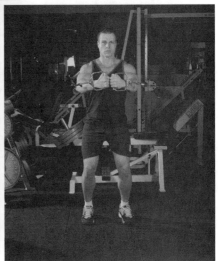

Push-up

The push-up exercise has become a neglected exercise that hasn't received the acclaim it warrants. The push-up is a very powerful exercise for developing the chest muscles, triceps and anterior deltoid muscles. It allows the trainee to utilize the proper biomechanics, which can better help isolate the chest muscles. Push-ups work beautifully in a super-set protocol, helping to fully exhaust the chest muscles for total recruitment of the muscle fibers in the chest.

Please notice the variation of hand widths that you can play with here. The wider the hand width, the more focus on the outer chest muscles. The closer the hand widths, as shown in the diamond hand position below, the more focus on the inner chest muscles and the triceps muscles of the arms.

PROPER ALIGNMENT

1. Align your body face down with your arms extended in an elevated position. Keep your elbows slightly bent.

2. The hands will be flat on the floor directly underneath and a little wider than shoulder width.

3. Keep the legs completely straight and your toes on the floor.

4. Throughout the exercise, keep your head looking down in a neutral position.

TECHNIQUE AND FORM

1. With your body properly aligned, lower yourself to within one inch of the floor. Ensure that your elbows travel out away from your body. Push-ups performed with the elbows traveling close to your body mainly target the triceps muscles.

2. Make sure to inhale through your nose on the way down and exhale through the mouth on your way up.

3. Focus on your chest muscles (feel them working here) and push your body off the floor using your toes as a pivot point.

4. Make sure to keep your back straight, stomach muscles tightened and keep your head in line with your body. Maintaining the proper alignment is crucial.

5. When you reach the top of the movement, make sure to contract the chest muscles as hard as you can. Try to avoid hyper-extending the elbow joints!

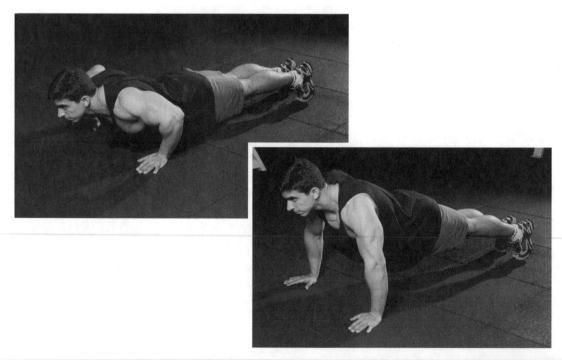

Push-up

Narrow hand width will hit more of the inner chest and tricep muscles.

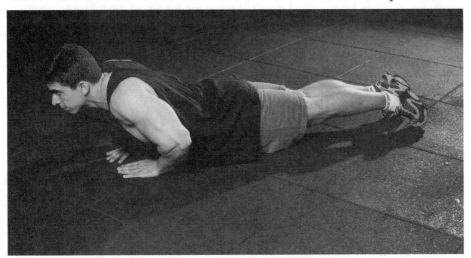

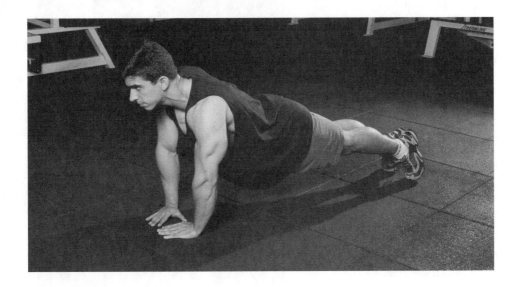

Assisted Push-up

If you need to, you may use this modified push-up exercise until you have gained enough strength to do the regular push-up. Take the same position and maintain the same form and technique as you would with the regular push-up. This time, however, let your knees stay in contact with the floor. You will find this exercise much easier because you will only be pushing up about half of your body weight. Follow the same procedure as the regular push-up.

If you can still not perform push-ups by using the modified position described above, then perform them standing up at an angle against the wall.

TECHNIQUE AND FORM

1. Take the same position and maintain the same form and technique as you would with the regular push-up. However, let your knees stay in contact with the floor.

2. You will find this exercise much easier because you will only be pushing up about half of your body weight.

3. Follow the same procedure as the regular push-up.

4. If you can still not perform push-ups by using the modified position described above, then perform them standing up at an angle against the wall.

MODIFICATIONS

Just as you can use various hand placement widths during the bench press exercise to focus in on specific areas of the chest, you can vary hand placement with the push-up.

• The wider your hand width, the more you'll zone in on the outer pecs with less triceps involvement.

• The closer the hand width, the more you'll zone in on the inner pecs with more triceps involvement.

• A medium hand width placement will be about 65 percent chest and 35 percent triceps.

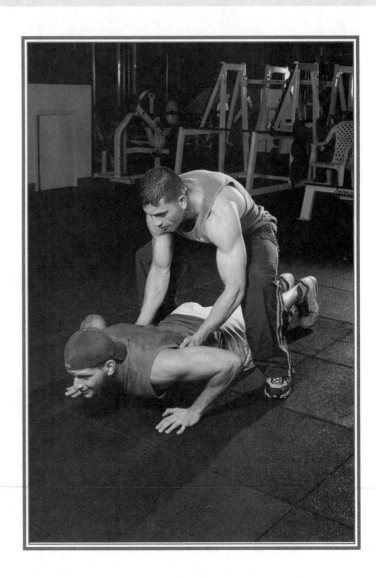

Assisted Push-up

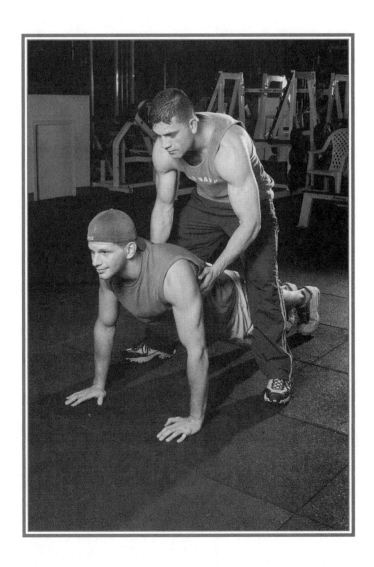

Chapter 9
Shoulders

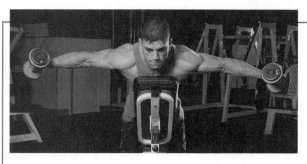

The shoulders are a beautiful muscle when properly developed. They provide an appearance of width and also give the illusion of bigger arms. In order to achieve the three dimensional look that shoulders provide, all three heads (anterior, medial and posterior) have to be developed.

The shoulders can be a very stubborn body part, especially if you don't know how to train them correctly. Even a slight variation in an exercise's proper form can mean the difference between no results and major results. Understand that most upper body exercises include the shoulders as a secondary muscle group, which could inhibit results for the shoulders because of over training. What it comes down to is this: If you don't learn how to train the shoulders correctly, you will not get the results you desire. If you learn what we teach below and implement the material into your shoulder training, you can definitely expect to receive the results you've desired.

THE BODY SCULPTING BIBLE FOR MEN

Dumbbell Shoulder Press

The dumbbell shoulder press will focus on all of the muscles of the shoulder with primary emphasis on the front and side deltoids. In addition, the upper part of the movement will also involve the triceps muscles. Again, the balancing act that dumbbells require makes this a challenging exercise that will give you the best return on your effort.

PROPER ALIGNMENT

1. Set your bench setting to a 90-degree angle (fully upright position), unless of course you already have access to a 90-degree angle seat.

2. Pick up your dumbbells and place them on your thighs.

3. Align your body from the bottom up.

4. Make sure that your feet are flat on the floor facing straight ahead throughout the exercise. Your knees should also be facing straight ahead.

5. Make sure that your whole back region is flush against the upright bench's back support. You must also concentrate on letting your chest relax. When you sit upright, it is natural that your chest will rise and move into the same upright position. This is bad because your chest muscles will end up becoming the primary muscles working during the exercise and will take the focus away from the shoulders. You want to focus on keeping your back straight against the back pad while completely relaxing your chest. This will help direct all of the stimulation onto shoulder muscles. If you see your chest rise or feel your chest muscles handling the majority of the work or helping to lift the weights, stop and cor-

rect yourself. You are either going too heavy or you just need to practice your form without weight. Once you are seated in a fully upright position with the dumbbells on your thighs, thrust up one leg at a time. Let momentum help to lift the dumbbells into your starting position.

6. Make sure that both dumbbells are held with your palms facing in front of you and level with the top of the shoulders.

7. Relax your chest while keeping your back totally upright and your head and neck as relaxed as possible. Please note that you must never turn your head while doing any of these exercises. Position your body into the proper alignment, keeping your head straight, and stay that way throughout the exercise. If you don't, you could end up seriously injured!

8. Keep your elbows as wide as possible as if you were trying to touch your elbows behind your back.

9. While keeping your upper arm horizontal to the floor, don't let the biceps and triceps sink below your shoulder height-this is the ideal level for a full range of motion for this exercise.

10. Keep your upper arms in a perpen-

dicular position while keeping your forearms pointed directly towards the ceiling at all times.

TECHNIQUE AND FORM

1. After you've set yourself up in proper alignment, slowly begin pressing the dumbbells up towards the ceiling in a smooth, controlled, fluid motion, making sure that you do not use any momentum. I advise that you do not touch the dumbbells at the top and instead press the weights in a straight-line overhead. Touching the dumbbells at the top of the movement may put some undue stress onto the rotator cuff muscles.

2. When you reach the top of the movement, do not lock out the elbow joint. When you lock out the elbow joint, you distribute all of the weight from the shoulders to the elbow joint, thus interrupting muscle stimulation. This can hurt the elbow joint and limit shoulder muscle stimulation.

3. Without resting, slowly bring the dumbbells back down, making sure that your arms are wide, your head is level and that you maintain an upright position with your chest relaxed.

Dumbbell Shoulder Press

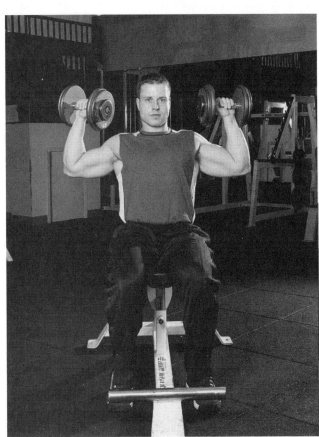

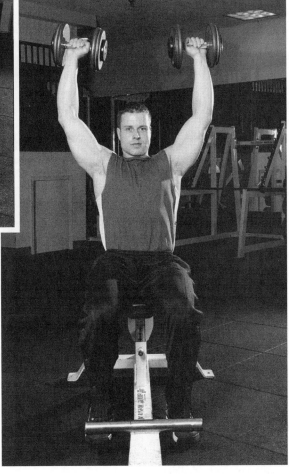

Dumbbell Lateral Raise

The dumbbell lateral raise is a superb isolation exercise that primarily targets the side deltoid. When performed correctly this exercise will add slabs of muscle to the medial head, providing you with extra inches of width. The key here is to leave the ego outside the gym: use a lower weight that allows you to concentrate on perfect form.

PROPER ALIGNMENT

1. Take a standing position with a shoulder-width stance. Align the body from the bottom up, beginning with the feet. Make sure the feet are pointing straight ahead.

2. Keep the knees pointing straight ahead and slightly bent to help avoid any unnecessary back strain.

3. Hold a dumbbell in each hand with arms down at your sides. Your palms should be pointed toward your body.

4. It is important to remember that as you lift the dumbbells, your palms should be facing downward, so your shoulder muscles rather than the biceps muscles do the work.

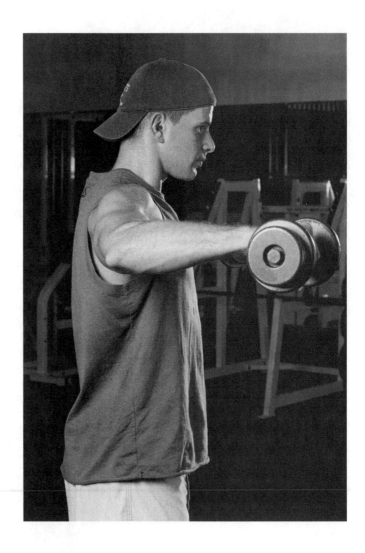

TECHNIQUE AND FORM

1. Keeping your arms straight and at the sides of your body, lift the weights directly out to the sides until they reach the level of your cheeks.

2. Hold the weights there for a one-second count.

3. While maintaining your posture and body alignment, slowly lower the dumbbells in a controlled fashion back to the starting point. Make sure you pick a dumbbell weight that allows you to practice perfect form. If you pick a weight that is too heavy, momentum will force muscles other than the shoulder to do the work. Some people have the tendency to bend at the elbows. Keeping the arms straight allows for better isolation of the medial deltoid.

Dumbbell Lateral Raise

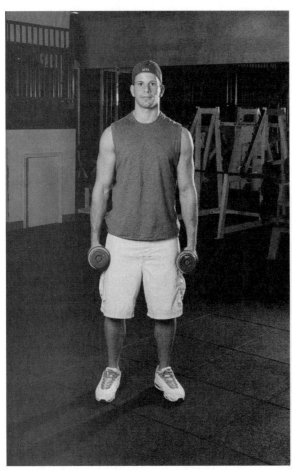

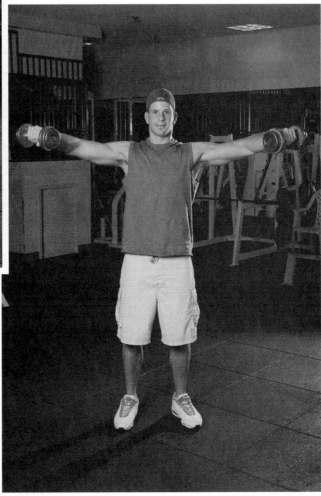

Military Press

Unlike behind-the-neck presses, which risk damaging the rotator cuffs, military presses are a great exercise to develop all three heads of the shoulder or deltoid muscles. You will find that a narrower grip focuses more on the muscles of the medial and rear deltoids with an emphasis on the triceps. The wider you go, the more you'll incorporate the front and medical deltoids. Make sure to use a light enough weigh to allow you a full range of motion; you should bring the bar down very close to your pec muscles of motion, they will see unbelievable results from their efforts.

PROPER ALIGNMENT

1. Take a seat on the military seat and place your feet flat on the floor in front of you. Your knees should also be facing straight ahead.

2. Take hold of the barbell with your grip of choice. Remember that grip variation will stimulate certain muscles more than others. The best thing you can do for your body is to assess your shoulder muscles and decide what portion of the three heads are in need of further development for overall muscle balance and symmetry.

3. Sit all the way back in the seat, making sure that your back is straight and flat against the back pad.

4. A mistake made when doing either this exercise or the dumbbell shoulder press is to stick the chest way out when pressing up. Do not do this! Remember, when you stick the chest out during the press, you take primary stimulation away from the shoulder muscles and direct it to the chest muscles. You want to relax the chest at all times during this exercise. If you see your chest rise or feel your chest muscles handling the majority of the work, stop and correct yourself. You may either be going too heavy, or you just need to practice your form without weight.

5. As you hold the bar, make sure that your arms and elbows are as wide as possible (as if you were trying to touch your elbows behind your back).

6. While keeping your upper arm horizontal to the floor, don't let the biceps and triceps region sink below shoulder height as this is the ideal level for a full range of motion for this exercise.

7. Keep your forearms in a perpendicular position (keeping your forearms pointed directly towards the ceiling at all times).

8. Make sure that your head and neck are as relaxed as possible throughout the entire exercise. Please note that you must never turn your head while doing any of these exercises. Position your body into the proper alignment, keeping your head straight, and stay that way throughout the exercise! If you don't, you could end up seriously injured.

TECHNIQUE AND FORM

Before you begin the exercise, close your eyes and visualize yourself doing the movement. Focus on the shoulder muscles you are about to stimulate. Remember what we discussed about assessing your shoulder muscles and comparing the balance and symmetry of the muscles. This goes for all muscles. Pay close attention to the muscles that are lagging behind others and concentrate all of your energies to those areas during the exercise. If your mus-

cles are already in balance and symmetric, focus on the muscle as a whole.

1. You should now be in position to begin. First, pick up the bar and begin the exercise from the top position.

2. With the arms and elbows wide and head level, slowly bring the bar down to an area slightly below the chin. The upper arm, from the elbow to the shoulder, should end up slightly below parallel to the floor, with your forearms perpendicular to the ceiling.

3. When you reach the bottom of the movement as your upper arms are lowered slightly below chin level slowly begin pressing upward in a smooth, controlled, fluid motion, without resting. Make sure that you do not use any momentum.

4. When you reach the top of the movement, do not lock out the elbow joint. When you lock out the elbow joint, you distribute all of the weight from the shoulders to the elbow joint, thus interrupting muscle stimulation. This can hurt the elbow joint and limit shoulder muscle stimulation.

5. From this point, slowly begin to lower the bar in a smooth, controlled, fluid motion, without resting.

Military Press

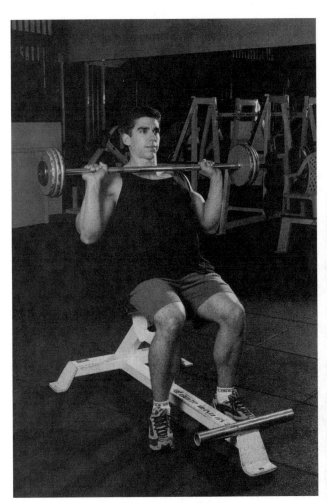

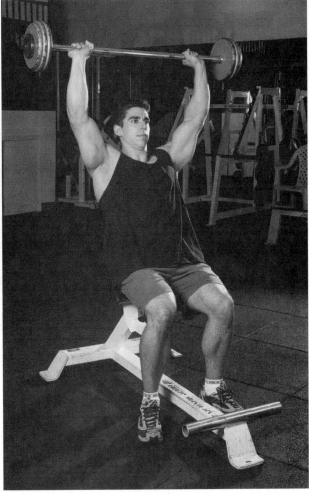

Upright Row

(Using A Cambered Bar Or Dumbbells)

Upright rows are a great exercise to develop the tie-in muscles, aesthetically tying your shoulders and trapezius muscles together and also for the medial head. You must make certain that you use very strict form with this exercise, avoiding momentum at all times. The rotator cuff muscles of the shoulder are extremely delicate and are prone to injuries that occur as a result of using poor form and excessive weight. The upright row exercise alone can stress the rotator cuff muscles. This makes it imperative that you use a weight you can handle using perfect form and technique with no momentum at all. We recommend that you practice the exercise using a cambered (E-Z Curl Bar) bar at first. This is usually much easier on the wrists and shoulders than a straight barbell. After you've mastered the perfect form methods, you can begin using two separate dumbbells for variety. We will now discuss the alignment phase of the exercise.

PROPER ALIGNMENT

1. Choose a weight for the cambered bar that is easy enough so you can focus only on your form. Once you have mastered the correct form, it will become second nature and you will find it easy to move up in weight, thereby being able to fully stimulate the shoulder muscles.

2. Grasp the bar using a shoulder-width grip.

3. Place your feet shoulder-width apart and point them straight ahead.

4. Keep your knees slightly bent at all times during the movement to take stress off the lower back region. Also, keep the knees pointing straight ahead.

5. Contract the abdominal muscles slightly to help keep your postural alignment.

6. Keep your back straight and body still as you do the exercise.

7. Relax the musculature of your chest and back.

8. Keep your head level and look straight ahead at all times during the exercise.

9. Hold the bar across your thighs and keep your palms facing toward your body.

10. Begin focusing on the muscles of the shoulder including the trapezius muscles. Although you will be pulling the weight up with your hands, you must let the elbows lead the motion, keeping them high as you pull up.

TECHNIQUE AND FORM

1. Before you begin the exercise, close your eyes and once again visualize yourself actually doing the movement while focusing on the shoulder and trapezius muscles.

2. With proper form and postural alignment, begin pulling the bar up slowly, concentrating on feeling the stimulation of the focused muscles.

3. Pull the bar up, leading with your elbows, to a point where it comes close to your chin.

4. The most important thing to do at this position of the exercise is to consciously focus on and physically contract the muscles of the trapezius.

5. Hold the contraction here for a count of one to two seconds.

6. With just enough time to contract the trap muscles, slowly begin lowering the bar while maintaining the same exact form and posture you did when pulling up.

7. When you reach the bottom (start) position, slowly begin pulling the bar back to the top position of the exercise using a smooth, controlled, fluid motion. Make sure that you do not jerk or use momentum to lift the bar at any time during this exercise.

Upright Row

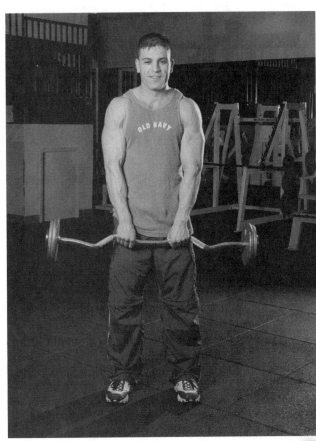

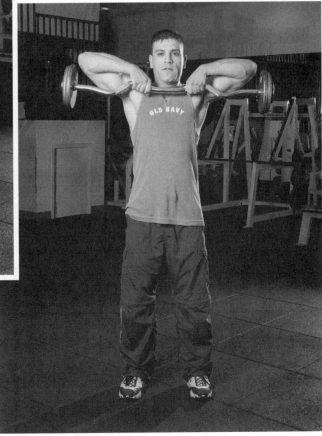

Bent-over Lateral Raise

The bent-over lateral raise is a great exercise for developing the rear deltoid muscles of the shoulder, which, in our opinion, is one of the most neglected muscles in the body. By using this exercise to develop this muscle, you will give your shoulders a fantastic three-dimensional look.

There are three ways that you can do this exercise. We will describe one in depth and the other two briefly. The first version is the seated bent-over lateral raise in which you sit on the edge of the bench, bend at the waist with your head down and lift the dumbbells to each side of your body. The other version is the standing bent-over lateral raise, in which you stand in the same postural alignment as you did with the standing dumbbell lateral raise with the exception that this time, you bend over at the hips. Once again, you will be bending your knees while keeping your back straight and parallel to the floor as you lift the dumbbells to the sides of your body, leading the movement with your elbows (this is the version to be used by those of you with little equipment).

The exercise we will discuss now, however, is the best exercise for developing the rear deltoids. This exercise is the bent-over lateral raise done on an incline bench. It will give you the best of both of the exercises we first discussed, allowing you to stay very strict while keeping you almost parallel to the floor. In addition, this exercise eliminates any stress to the lower back.

PROPER ALIGNMENT

1. Choose two light dumbbells so that you may practice perfect form.

2. Rest your entire torso, from your pelvic bone to your chest, on the incline bench's angled pad with your head and eyes looking straight ahead.

3. Position your feet shoulder-width apart, pointing them straight ahead at all times during the exercise.

4. Make sure that your knees are bent so there is no unnecessary lower back stress.

5. Bring the dumbbells down to each side of your body with your palms facing each other.

6. Make sure that you are positioned steadily on the bench incline.

7. Bring your head up to the level of your torso, which must be close to or parallel to the floor. Look straight ahead.

8. As you prepare to do the exercise, focus all of your attention and concentration on the rear deltoid muscles of the shoulder. Know where these mus-cles are located and how they feel when stimulated. This is why we suggest that you go light, so that you may isolate these muscles without incorporating others into the movement.

9. As you lift the dumbbells to the sides of your body, your elbows will be leading the motion. Many people who do this and similar exercises lead the movement with the dumbbells and take all of the focus off the shoulders. When you lead the exercise movement with the dumbbells, you will not opti-mally stimulate the desired rear deltoid muscles.

TECHNIQUE AND FORM

1. Slowly and without momentum, begin lifting the dumbbells out to each side of your body.

2. Try to move your whole arm together, or at least make sure that the elbows are leading the movement.

3. Do not lift your torso as you lift. If you find that you are in fact lifting for momentum assistance, stop! Either lighten the weight or rest for one minute and do your next set. Don't just go through the motions only concerned with getting the weights up. Focus on isolation of the rear deltoid muscles, and make them work hard.

4. Make sure that you lift the dumb-bells straight out to your sides rather than behind you. This is very important for rear deltoid isolation.

5. Maintain your postural alignment and bring the dumbbells up to level with your shoulders or slightly higher.

6. Squeeze the dumbbells back while you contract the rear deltoid muscles as hard as you can. Hold this contrac-tion for one second.

7. From this point, slowly begin lower-ing the dumbbells, making sure that you make the rear deltoid muscles con-tinue to work during the lowering por-tion of the exercise.

8. As you reach the bottom (start) posi-tion, do not rest. Once again, slowly begin lifting the dumbbells out to each side of your body in a smooth, con-trolled and fluid motion, without using momentum.

Bent-over Lateral Raise

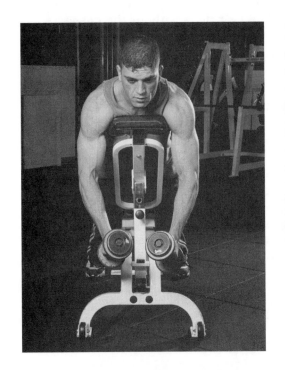

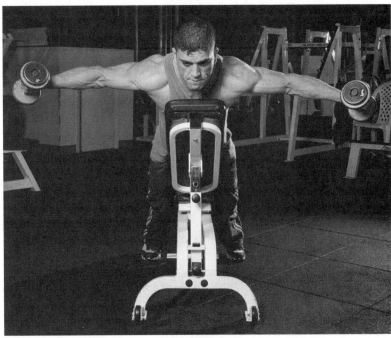

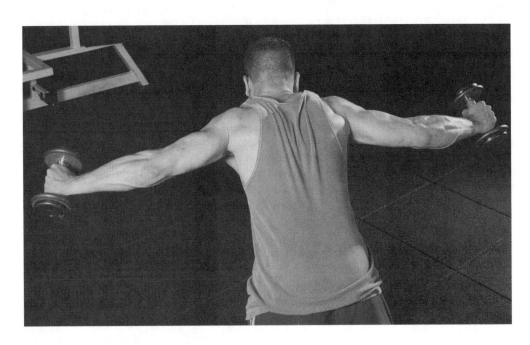

Seated Rear-delt Machine

The seated rear-delt machine is a great exercise to use for variety in your shoulder training arsenal. It will give you the ability to really focus on isolating the rear delts without the possibility of lower back injury and the burden of having to bend over at the hips. This is a perfect exercise for those who feel dizzy when bent over or feel too much chest compression from having to lean on the incline bench, or have lower back problems.

PROPER ALIGNMENT

1. Seat yourself on the machine and position your body so that you are sitting upright with your chest flush against the vertical pad. There should be a seat adjustment that will allow you to raise and lower the seat. Bring the seat to a height where your chin can rest neutrally on the edge of the pad in front of you. This is a good height to optimize the proper anatomical position for this shoulder exercise.

2. Keep your feet flat on the floor and pointing straight ahead during the movement. Also, keep your knees pointing straight ahead at all times. On most rear-delt machines, you will find inner thigh pads for added stability. Keep your thighs snug against the pads to give you the added support needed to secure your core musculature.

3. This machine is often used as a pec deck and gives you the option of adjusting the arm bars to your liking. For this particular exercise, you will want the arm bars brought to the back position so they are just about touching one another. You also might have the option of taking your handgrip in a palms facing position or an over-hand position. Take the overhand position since this will take much stress off the wrists and allow better muscle control and isola-tion of the rear shoulders, thus negating the triceps muscles as much as possible from the movement.

4. Make sure that you keep a slight bend in the elbows at all times. This bend of the arms will help make sure that you keep the focus of resistance on the rear delts and off the triceps. You might reach a level of fatigue where you are forced to use the triceps muscles to move the weight. When you reach this point, either resist the temptation or simply lower the weight.

5. Keep your chest cavity against the chest pad at all times during the exercise with your torso totally upright.

TECHNIQUE AND FORM

1. Begin the exercise with your feet flat on the floor, thighs pinned snug against the thigh pads, and body upright with chest against the pad and chin rested on the edge.

2. With hands holding the grips in an overhand position, make sure that your elbows are pointed directly out to the sides. This is very important for isola-tion of the rear delt muscles.

3. Before you begin the movement, make sure you are consciously focused on the rear delt muscles and begin to isometrically contract them before moving the weight. This might take some practice to perfect, but you will soon multiply your muscle isolation abilities ten-fold.

4. Begin bringing the bars away from each other and maintain your anatomi-cal positioning at all times. Bring the bars as far back as possible without jerking or using momentum to do so.

5. As you reach the top of the movement, with arms fully extended out-wards, try to hold this position for one count while feeling the rear shoulder muscles taking the brunt of the resis-tance. At this point, really squeeze the rear delts.

6. Slowly allow the arms to return to the start position, resisting the bars on the negative portion of the exercise.

7. Once you have reached the position where the bars are just about touching each other, do not allow the weight stack to touch the bottom. You want to keep constant tension on the muscles and must stop right before the weights touch bottom. From here immediately begin to bring the bars apart once again with great form.

Seated Rear-delt Machine

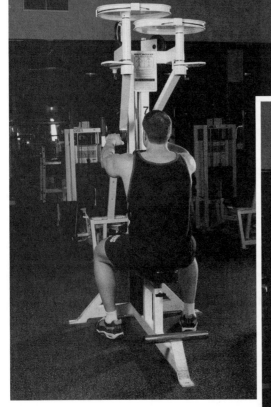

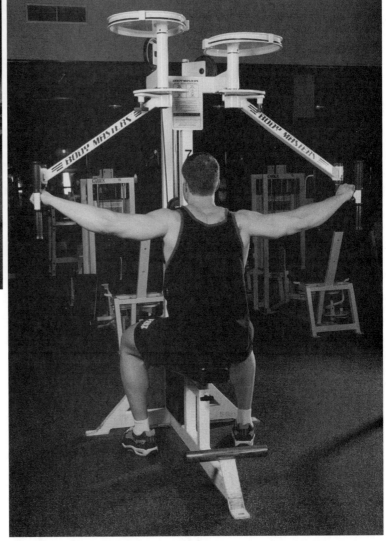

Chapter 10
Triceps

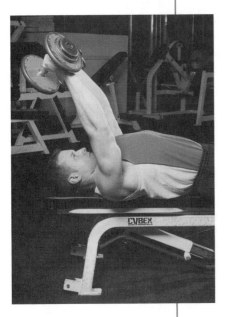

The triceps muscle, located on the back of the upper arm, is a three-headed muscle with a horseshoe appearance that requires different angles of training for full development. A lot of people don't realize that just one exercise for most body parts simply won't cut it, unless you want a simple looking body with simple looking muscles. Specific exercises will stimulate specific muscles to work primarily and incorporate other muscles to work as the secondary muscles.

While most guys that want big arms usually focus on the biceps, 2/3 of the arm size is provided by the triceps! Therefore, if you want big arms, you cannot afford to neglect the triceps. The following exercises incorporate all angles of training, providing total triceps muscle development.

10

THE **BODY**
SCULPTING
BIBLE
FOR**MEN**

Overhead Dumbbell Extension

(Using one dumbbell supported by two hands)

The overhead dumbbell extension focuses on the middle and inner heads of the triceps muscles. You can do this exercise either while seated or while standing. We recommend you do it seated as you will be less likely to cheat using momentum. One very important thing to remember with this exercise is to keep the elbows pointed to the ceiling above you at all times during the movement. This will help create a full range of motion for the triceps. You also need to hold the upper arms close to your head as you extend the weight overhead. Finally, one of the most important things to remember and perfect with this exercise is your handgrip on the dumbbell. It is not easy to get a perfectly even grip for both hands with this exercise. If you fail to grip the dumbbell evenly, you may end up directing the force of the dumbbell resistance to one arm more than the other. This will create muscle imbalance between the two muscles. To fix this, you must learn to either grip the top, inner portion of the dumbbell with a separate even grip for both hands or with an overlapping grip having one hand overlap the other. We recommend that you choose, if available, a dumbbell that adequately allows two separate and even handgrips. Unfortunately, most dumbbells will not allow a great deal of space to securely grip in this fashion. In this case, you must learn to perfect your overlapping grip for better balance and muscle symmetry.

PROPER ALIGNMENT

1. Choose a weight that you believe to be light enough to practice perfect form. Place the dumbbell on top of your thigh. You can also have someone hand the dumbbell to you from behind. This is especially useful when using very heavy weight and to avoid injuring the shoulder joints.

2. Sit on a bench with a 90-degree angled back pad.

3. Sit all the way back into the seat, making sure that your back is flat against the pad at all times during the movement.

4. Before lifting the weight into position overhead, make sure that your feet are placed flat on the floor and pointed straight ahead. Make sure that your knees are also pointing straight ahead. Keep the head level and facing straight ahead at all times during the movement.

5. Position the dumbbell overhead or have someone hand it to you from behind. Grasp the dumbbell with your grip of choice.

6. Point your elbows straight to the ceiling above you while holding your arms and elbows close to your head for triceps isolation.

TECHNIQUE AND FORM

1. With the dumbbell overhead and in position, begin lowering the dumbbell while keeping the elbows pointed directly to the ceiling. It is important to do this because it will help isolate the triceps muscle and provide a full range of productive motion. It will also help you avoid hitting the dumbbell on the back of your head while extending and lowering the dumbbell.

2. As you lower the dumbbell, focus on the triceps muscle and feel the stretch. Always take this negative portion slow and stay in control.

3. Lower the dumbbell to a point where your forearms are slightly below parallel to the ground. You should feel a big stretch in the triceps.

4. Without any rest and avoiding the use of momentum, begin pressing the weight back up to the top position. Make sure that you are using perfect form, while maintaining the correct postural alignment.

5. All of your attention must be on the triceps muscle, focusing on the isolation of the muscles.

6. As you approach the top of the movement, contract the triceps muscles as hard as you possibly can while avoiding intensely locking out the elbow joints.

7. Hold this contraction for a 1-2 second count and begin your descent, lowering the dumbbell in a slow, controlled and fluid manner.

Overhead Dumbbell Extension

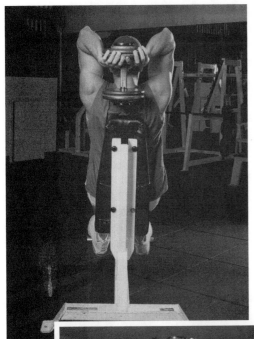

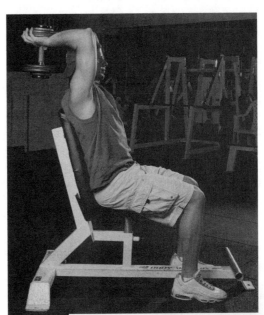

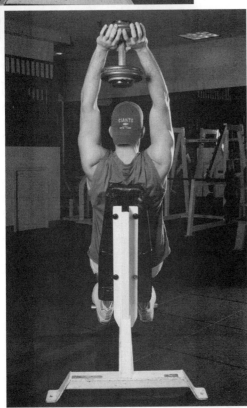

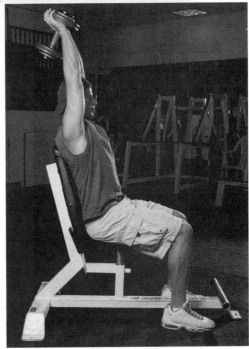

Lying Dumbbell Extension

(Using two dumbbells simultaneously)

This exercise is a one of our favorites (second only to triceps dips). The lying position provides greater stability to lift more safely, preventing a chance of injury to your lower back. It also allows greater leverage to occur, much like the flat dumbbell press, allowing better strength output with a smoother exercise movement. Always make sure to move the dumbbells slowly from start to finish and squeeze the triceps muscles at the top of the movement to really feel the triceps working.

PROPER ALIGNMENT

1. Pick up two dumbbells, making sure that they are light enough for you to practice perfect form or for simply warming up your triceps muscles.

2. Sit at the end of a flat bench with the weights positioned upright on top of your thighs.

3. It is very important to grip both dumbbell handles all the way at the end closest to your thighs. Make sure to slide your hands all the way to the bottom of the handle so that the pinky side of your hand is up against the weight plate. Doing this will help you control the weight better while also allowing you to contract the triceps muscles harder at the top of the movement.

4. Thrust each dumbbell up just as you would when doing a dumbbell bench press.

5. Lay back on the bench and place your feet flat onto the floor.

6. As you are lying down, keeping the long side of the dumbbells and the palms of your hands facing each other at all times, press the weights up using your chest muscles (chest press). You

will begin the exercise in this position to avoid stressing the elbow joint. If you start at the bottom position of this exercise, you can easily create too much pressure on the elbow joint capsule, risking long-term injury. Remember, throughout the movement, the palms of your hands and your inner elbows must always face each other. You want to make sure that your whole arm is in a direct line with your front shoulder (anterior deltoid).

7. You must also make sure that your elbows are pointing directly at the ceiling at all times during the exercise.

8. Begin the exercise with the arms fully extended overhead, holding the dumbbells high to the ceiling.

TECHNIQUE AND FORM

1. Once you are in the proper body alignment with the dumbbells overhead, slowly lower the dumbbells down toward your shoulders. While doing this, your elbows will remain pointing directly at the ceiling; and your entire arm from the elbows to the shoulders is frozen at all times. These steps are necessary for proper triceps stimulation

during this exercise. Remember to consciously focus all of your attention on proper form and stimulation of the triceps muscles.

2. As you lower the dumbbells, stop just before the dumbbells reach your shoulders and begin to slowly and smoothly extend your arms from the elbows to the hands back up to the starting position of the exercise. Remember to keep your upper arm frozen in place.

3. As you reach the top of the exercise, contract the triceps muscles as hard as you possibly can for complete muscle stimulation. Make sure that you avoid excessively locking the elbow joint. Once you reach the position of full elbow extension, do not thrust the elbow joint into a locked position. Instead, contract the triceps muscles as hard as you possibly can. Practice using light weights with this technique as practice will make for perfect execution of the exercise and better results. Also, make sure that there is a smooth transition when switching directions from lowering the dumbbells to raising the dumbbells. Do not rest between lowering and raising the dumbbell.

Lying Dumbbell Extension

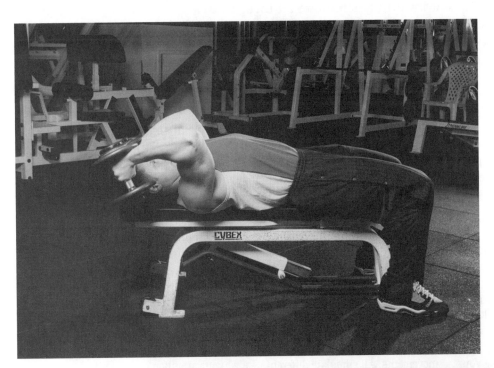

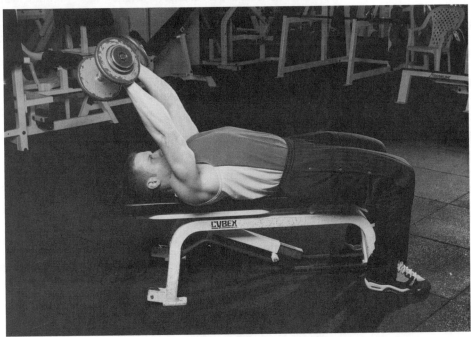

Lying E-Z Bar Extension

This triceps exercise is one that will fully stimulate all three muscles of the triceps. It is performed with an E-Z curl bar, a curved bar usually found in the free weight section of your gym or health club. If you don't have access to this type of bar, just stick with the Lying Dumbbell Triceps Extensions, as they are both very similar to one another. You can also use this exercise to build your strength and coordination in preparation for the Lying Dumbbell Triceps Extensions.

PROPER ALIGNMENT

1. Set up a cambered bar (E-Z curl bar) with some light weight on each side or get one that is already pre-weighted. You can rest the curl bar on your thighs and lay back, set it in place so that it is at the base of your head while you lie down, or simply have someone hand it to you when you are already lying down.

2. Before lifting the bar or having it handed to you, lay back on the bench and place your feet flat onto the floor, pointing straight ahead.

3. As you are lying down, lift the bar into place by pressing it up using your chest muscles (like the chest press). Hold it up above your head and stay there. You will begin the exercise in this position to avoid stressing the elbow joint. If you start at the bottom position of this exercise, you can easily create too much pressure on the elbow joint capsule, risking long-term injury. Once you begin the movement from the top, the pressure in the elbow joints will be reduced as you reach the bottom position.

4. Remember, the palms of your hands and inner elbows must always face each other during the exercise.

5. Make sure that your whole arm is in a direct line with your front shoulder (anterior deltoid).

6. This exercise will be done slightly different from the lying two-dumbbell extension. Take a grip on the bar and position your hands about 8 to 10 inches apart; bring the E-Z bar overhead and position your elbows so that they are pointing directly to the ceiling above you but now, you will point your elbows slightly behind you and toward the ceiling on an angle. Doing this with the E-Z curl bar in your hands will automatically distribute the resistance from resting on the elbow joints to the triceps muscles instead. We don't recommend that you do this with the lying dumbbell extension because the two movements will stimulate different areas of the triceps muscles.

Begin the exercise just as we described it to you and maintain that technique, form and postural alignment throughout the exercise.

TECHNIQUE AND FORM

1. Once you are in the proper body alignment with the E-Z curl bar overhead, slowly begin to lower the bar down toward your forehead. While doing this, your elbows will remain pointing slightly behind you on an angle toward the ceiling.

2. Make sure that your entire arm from the elbows to your shoulders is frozen in place at all times during the exercise. These steps are necessary for proper triceps stimulation during this exercise.

3. Remember to consciously focus all of your attention on proper form and stimulation of the triceps muscles.

4. As you lower the bar, stop just before it reaches your forehead and begin to slowly and smoothly extend your arms back up to the starting position of the exercise.

5. As you reach the top of the exercise, make sure you are consciously contracting the triceps muscles as hard as you possibly can for complete muscle stimulation.

6. Hold this contraction for one second.

7. Make sure there is a smooth transition when switching directions. There should be no rest at all when switching from the bottom position to the upward extension of the bar.

Lying E-Z Bar Extension

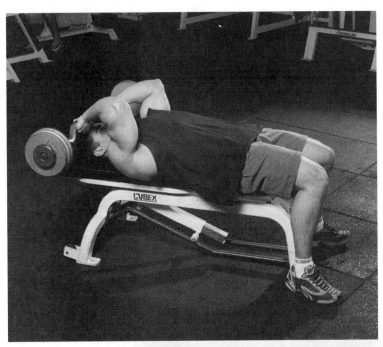

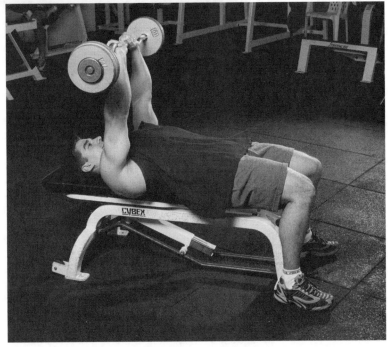

Triceps Dip

The triceps dip is a great muscle-enhancing exercise focusing on the lower triceps, which are closer to the elbow. There is a major difference between the triceps dip and the chest dip. When we discussed the chest dips, we told you to bend at the knees, lock your feet and bend forward as you lower yourself. You must stay bent over to keep the focus of resistance in the chest muscles. But with the triceps dip we are trying to isolate the triceps muscles and instead avoid stimulation of the chest muscles. To do this you will need a dip station or machine. If you are working out in your home, you can purchase an inexpensive dip unit from one of the sports-related retail chains or a wholesale fitness supply store.

PROPER ALIGNMENT

1. First, place your hands on the parallel bars as you position yourself for postural alignment. The best way to do this is to raise yourself up onto the dip bars by locking out your arms. Align your body starting with your head and moving down to your feet. We have found a fantastic way of doing triceps dips that makes it very easy to isolate the triceps muscles. To make it as easily understood as possible, your entire body from head to toes should be as straight as possible throughout the exercise.

2. As you lower yourself from the lockout position, keep your head in a neutral or level position.

3. Your chest and shoulders must be completely upright and as straight as possible.

4. Your arms and elbows will ride close to your body as you lower yourself and when pushing to triceps lockout.

5. Your abdominal muscles should be contracted slightly to hold you in position.

6. Your legs must be completely straight, and your feet flat as if you were standing up. Now, don't think that because the setup is easy, the exercise will be easily executed. Yes, the set-up for the exercise is easier than most; but this easy set up makes the triceps isolation and stimulation incredibly powerful.

TECHNIQUE AND FORM

1. As you lower yourself down, you lean back to help hold your body in the upright position.

2. Lower yourself slowly while resisting your bodyweight all the way to the bottom position.

3. Keep the elbows close to your body, helping to better isolate the triceps muscles.

4. Keeping your legs straight and feet flat to the floor, lower yourself to the floor. You can do two things here: You can either stop lowering your body right before your feet touch, or you can lower yourself to the point where you tap your feet flat on the ground and immediately begin your return upward. We prefer the latter since we know that when we tap bottom, we have completed the full range of motion for complete muscle stimulation and should explode into the upward press. Some people will not be tall enough to touch their feet at the bottom of the training apparatus being used. Also, you would never want to lower yourself to a point where you could injure yourself just to touch your feet flat on the floor. There is such a point! In any of these cases, just lower your body until your upper arms (from your elbows to your shoulders) are parallel to the floor. Then, immediately begin your return upward.

5. No matter what technique you use at the bottom position, after you've

reached that point, slowly and with a smooth transition begin to press your body upward, maintaining your upright posture.

6. As you begin pressing upward, make sure that all of your focus is directed to your triceps muscles. This alone will help stimulate the triceps by increased muscle control and as a reminder to maintain proper alignment.

7. As you near the top of the motion, your goal is not to lock the joint but instead to contract and squeeze the triceps muscles as hard as you possibly can for a 1-2 second count. It is important to let the triceps muscles hold you in this position rather than lock the elbow joints. Otherwise, you can injure the joint plus you take all of the resistance off the triceps muscles and put it onto the joints and bones. Remember that there should be no rest at the top of the exercise after the contraction period. From that lockout position, once again slowly lower yourself back to the bottom position as you resist the weight of your body. If you get to a point where your body weight is too light for the exercise, you may use a dip belt to hook some additional weight to your body, thus increasing the resistance. Please make sure that if you do use additional weight, you do so in incremental stages.

Triceps Dip

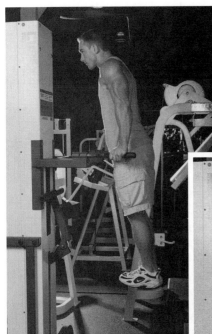

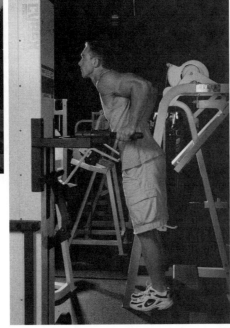

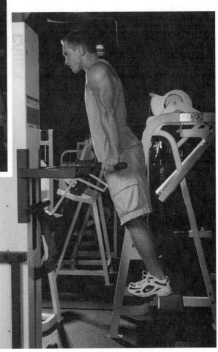

Bench Dip

Triceps Dips can also be performed between benches if you are unable to perform them on the parallel bars, for whatever reason. Just like parallel bar triceps dips, this exercise will primarily focus on all three heads of the triceps. We guarantee you that this exercise will help you achieve those big and ripped horseshoe triceps that you are looking for, thus adding inches to your arm girth. Remember, triceps make up 2/3 of the arm size so neglecting them is not a good idea. This is a great exercise for developing the strength necessary to do the Triceps Dips exercise on the parallel dip bar unit.

PROPER ALIGNMENT

1. Place two benches in parallel to each other (side by side) with sufficient space in between them to allow for your palms of the hands to be on one bench and the back of your feet on top of the other bench.

2. Sit between the two benches with your palms on the bench behind you and with your legs on top of the other bench. If you are aligned correctly, your body should resemble an L.

TECHNIQUE AND FORM

1. Use the strength of your triceps to lower you towards the ground in a gradual and controlled movement.

2. Continue to lower yourself until the upper arm and the forearms create a 90 degree angle.

3. Use your triceps to push yourself back up to the starting position.

Important Notes

1. Once again guys, leave the ego outside of the gym. Do not move up and down in a jerky or uncontrolled manner as this exercise can place extreme stress on the shoulder girdle.

2. If unable to perform this exercise, you may use a partner's assistance to support part of your weight.

3. As you get stronger, you may want to have a partner put plates on top of your quadriceps muscles as illustrated in the picture at right. However, ensure that the partner is always there providing weight stability and also ensure that the weight is never placed on top of the knee joint.

Bench Dip

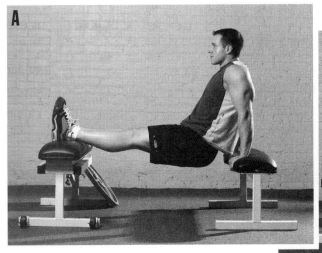

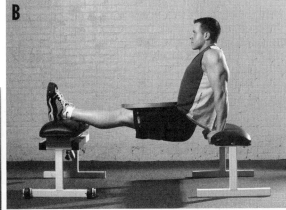

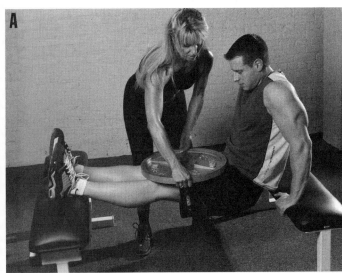

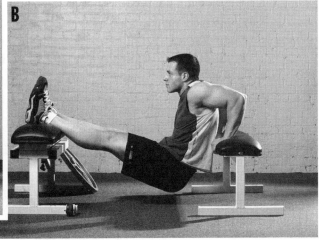

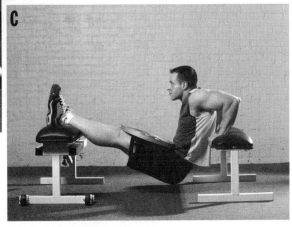

E-Z Curl Bar Close-Grip Press

This exercise can be done one of two ways. It can be done alone as a triceps and inner chest exercise or as a secondary superset exercise with the E-Z Bar Triceps Extension exercise. We will explain this exercise in detail, and how you incorporate it will depend on the phase of training you have reached. The conventional way to do the close-grip bench press would be with a barbell. It also calls for the arms to widen at the bottom, putting more emphasis on the inner chest muscles than the triceps. Our version of this exercise will obviously be done with the E-Z curl bar and with a different arm position than the conventional version. This puts emphasis on the triceps with a secondary workload to the inner chest muscles.

PROPER ALIGNMENT

This exercise will incorporate many of the same alignment positions as the Lying E-Z Bar Triceps Extension exercise

1. Set up the E-Z bar with some weight or get one that is pre-weighted. You can rest the bar on your thighs and bring it back overhead, set it in place so that it is at the base of your head while you lie down, or simply have someone hand it to you when you are already lying down.

2. Before lifting the bar or having it handed to you, lay back on the bench and place your feet flat onto the floor, pointing straight ahead.

3. As you are lying down lift the bar into place by pressing it up using your chest muscles (just like the chest press). Hold it above your head and stay there. You will begin the exercise in this position to avoid stressing the elbow joint.

4. Remember to make sure that your whole arm is in direct line with your front shoulder (anterior deltoid). Your arms must stay close to your body and follow in a straight line from shoulder, to elbow, to arm. This is what will create primary isolation on the triceps muscles and allow better control of the bar.

5. Take a position on the bar so that your hands are in the outer curved position of the bar. The inner curved position will create too much wrist strain. The proper width will be about 8-10 inches apart.

TECHNIQUE AND FORM

1. Once you are in the proper alignment with the E-Z curl bar overhead, slowly begin to lower the bar down as if you were lowering the bar during a bench press movement. But remember, your arms will now stay close to your body with your front shoulders and arms in a straight line.

2. As you lower the bar, keep your arms riding closely to the sides of your body. This technique is essential for proper triceps stimulation.

3. Remember to consciously focus all of your attention on proper form and intense stimulation of the triceps during the movement.

4. As you continue to lower the bar, do so in a controlled manner and bring the bar down to around mid-chest. Without resting, and without momentum, use your triceps muscles to push the bar off your chest and back to the start position. Remember to maintain your proper form with the arms riding close to the sides of your body.

5. As you reach the top of the movement, squeeze the triceps muscles as hard as you can without locking out your elbow joints.

6. Hold this contraction for 1 second.

7. Make sure that there is a smooth transition when switching directions from the top position going into the lowering of the bar, and also from the bottom position going into the extension or raising of the bar. There should be no rest at all when switching from the bottom position into the upward extension of the bar.

E-Z Curl Bar Close-Grip Press

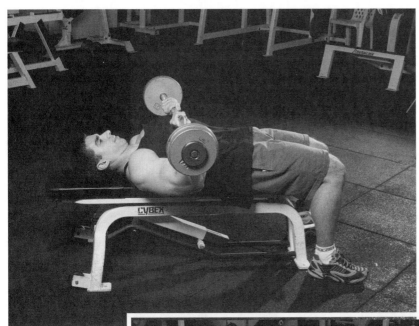

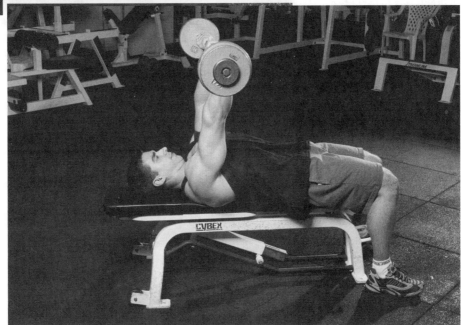

Close-Grip Dumbbell Press

The Close-Grip Dumbbell Press is an excellent compound movement that not only targets the triceps muscle hard but also, as a bonus, targets the middle of your chest. The alignment used for this exercise is the same as the alignment used for chest exercises with the exception that you will need to retract the scapula in order to bring the chest above the shoulders.

TECHNIQUE AND FORM

1. With the dumbbells on your thighs, thrust one leg up, leveraging one dumbbell up to around your chest level.

2. Immediately thrust the second dumbbell upward while simultaneously allowing momentum and the dumbbells to guide you back into the lying position; use your abdominal muscles to help safely ease you into position.

3. Lay back and align your body using the alignment instructions presented for chest exercises but retracting the scapula to bring the chest above the shoulders.

4. Once you are in position, instead of bringing the dumbbells to the outside of the chest, hold them close to your chest. The handles of the dumbbells and palms of your hands must face each other with the elbows riding close to your body during movement. Your forearms must be perpendicular to the ceiling during the entire exercise. This close-grip movement will stimulate the inner chest muscles while a primary emphasis will be delivered to the triceps muscles as well.

5. Because your shoulder muscles are more likely to move the weight than your chest muscles, you must retract the shoulder blades back or together against the flat bench. This slight variation will take the shoulders out of the chest movement, allowing the chest and triceps muscles to be the primary muscles working during the exercise.

6. With the chest in its elevated position, the elbows out and wide and the forearms perpendicular to the floor, press the dumbbells up toward the ceiling.

7. As you press the weight up, put your mind into the chest and triceps muscles by concentrating on and feeling the muscles contract as you push upward.

8. As you reach the top of the exercise, you must continue to consciously focus on the targeted muscles while physically contracting these muscles as hard as you possibly can. Your goal is to get the most intense contraction possible in the top position!

9. In this position, squeeze and hold for a count of 1-2 seconds.

10. Slowly begin lowering the weight while holding proper postural alignment throughout the exercise.

11. As the dumbbells are lowered to the start position, they should touch your chest. This allows for a full stretch of the chest and triceps muscles.

12. Without rest, slowly begin to press the dumbbells up again in a controlled, smooth, fluid motion, without using any momentum.

Close-Grip Dumbbell Press

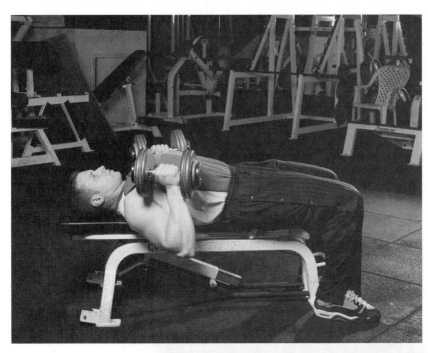

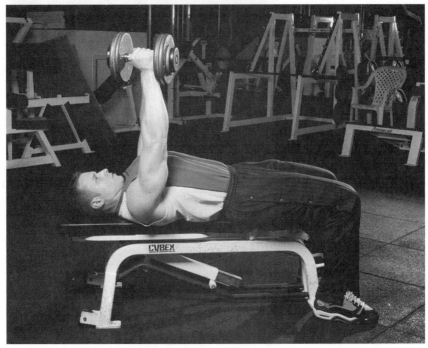

Triceps Pushdowns

This exercise often is performed incorrectly. Some common mistakes include the following:

1. Too much bending at the hips, which incorporates chest muscle activity. Proper form for this exercise means staying as straight as possible with a very slight bend to prevent lower back injury.

2. Bending over with the cable set on one side of the head. This causes the crucial balance of the resistance to be thrown off because force is greater at one side of the body than the other. Many professional trainers and athletes do this all the time. For proper form, keep the cable right at the center of your body.

3. Allowing the arms to come up during the negative portion of the exercise. Proper form calls for the upper arms (from the elbows to the shoulder) to stay locked at the sides of the body and remain there until the end of the exercise, when you have to return to the start position. Only the forearms should move.

This is a great exercise if done correctly. Follow the proper form and techniques and you will soon have the fat free and firm triceps you desire.

PROPER ALIGNMENT

You have the option of using a v-bar, a short cambered bar attachment, a rope, or a straight bar attachment for this exercise. Choose the bar that gives you the most comfortable grip. You can also change bars over time in order to add variety to your program.

1. Stand in front of the cable and take hold of the bar. Bring the bar down by bringing your arms (from the elbow to the shoulder) to the sides of your body and lock them there.

2. Position your feet shoulder width apart with your feet pointing straight ahead.

3. Slightly bend your knees and keep your torso upright throughout the movement.

4. Keep your head pointing straight ahead and avoid looking down; otherwise you will tend to bend over.

TECHNIQUE AND FORM

1. Holding the bar with your arms positioned in place at your sides, begin by isometrically contracting the triceps muscles before moving the bar down.

2. Begin pushing the bar down while keeping your elbows pinned to your sides.

3. Push down until you have reached full extension. Avoid locking the elbow joint out hard. Make sure you squeeze the triceps muscles as hard as you possibly can at lockout. You are to focus on squeezing the triceps muscles hard, not the elbow joint. There is a major difference that practice will perfect.

4. When you've reached the bottom position, squeeze the triceps muscles and hold for a count of 1 second.

5. Begin to allow the bar to rise while maintaining your posture and arms at the sides.

6. Let the bar come up to the point where your forearms are slightly higher than parallel to the floor. At this point, without resting, begin once again pushing down to the bottom position.

7. Follow this form throughout this exercise and your triceps will burn with delight. If you continue with this proper alignment, technique and form, your triceps will very soon develop into arms of beauty!

Triceps Pushdowns

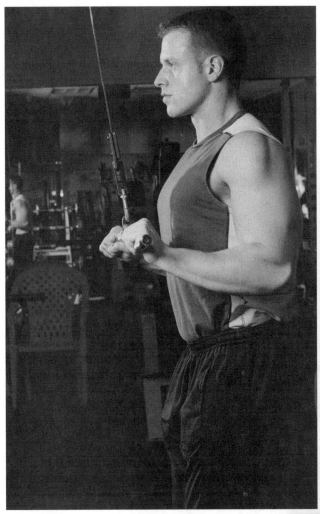

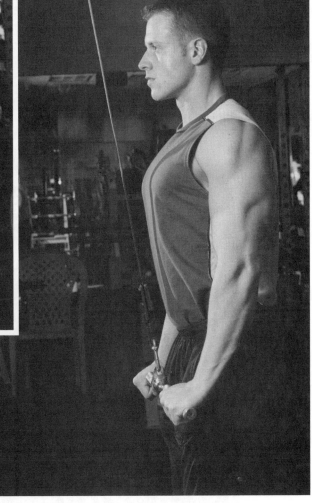

Triceps Kickback

This is a great isolation exercise if you settle for using lighter weights and just concentrate on using good form. Sloppy or incorrect technique will not allow you to get any benefit out of this exercise. This exercise will provide you with a killer contraction at the top of the movement. Try to hold that contraction for a second or two in order to really fry those triceps!

PROPER ALIGNMENT

1. With this exercise, you will be training one arm at a time. Starting with the right triceps, lean down on a flat bench and place your left knee and your left hand on the bench for support. Your right leg will remain in a semi-straight position, with the foot flat on the floor. Maintain a flat back throughout the exercise.

2. Pick up a dumbbell with the right hand using an overhand grip, making sure that the weight is light enough to maintain proper form throughout the exercise.

3. In the bent-over position, place the upper arm (right humerus) flush against the right side of your body. Make sure to allow your lower arm to remain loose.

4. Take note that when you are ready to begin this exercise the upper and lower arm of the triceps should form a 90-degree angle.

5. Reverse the same protocol when training the left triceps.

TECHNIQUE AND FORM

1. Once again, make sure that the lower and upper arm are at a 90-degree angle, and the dumbbell is held with an overhand grip.

2. Begin the exercise by extending the lower arm back until it is at full extension.

3. Make sure that you keep the upper arm pressed against the right side of the body during the exercise.

4. Once the elbow reaches the point of full extension, contract the triceps as hard as possible. Make sure to avoid hyperextension of the elbow.

5. Slowly lower the dumbbell back to the 90-degree angle.

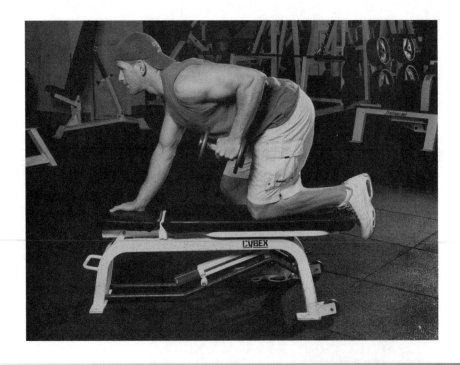

Triceps Kickback

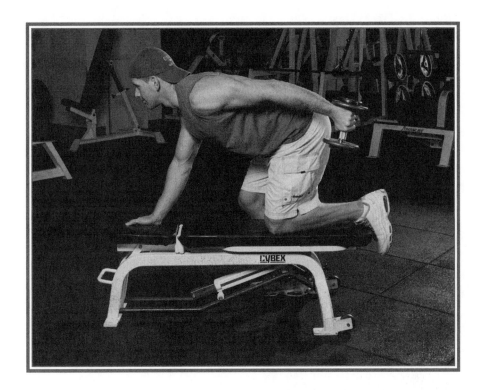

Chapter 11
Biceps

The biceps muscles are located on the front of the upper arms and are a two-headed muscle that serves to lift the forearms upwards. Biceps are probably one of the simplest muscles to train. However, just like chest muscles, you can go to any gym in the country and probably see that 90 percent of the people training them are using incorrect form.

11

THE**BODY SCULPTING BIBLE** FOR**MEN**

Dumbbell Curl

(Using two dumbbells simultaneously, while standing)

The dumbbell biceps curl is a great exercise for building the biceps muscles. We suggest that you do this exercise standing up and supporting yourself against a wall for good body mechanics and strict form.

PROPER ALIGNMENT

The dumbbell biceps curl is a great exercise for building the biceps muscles. We suggest that you do this exercise standing up and supporting yourself against a wall for good body mechanics and strict form.

1. Choose two light dumbbells so that you can practice perfect form.

2. With the dumbbells in hand, begin the alignment of your body by placing your feet about shoulder width apart with the feet pointing straight ahead of you.

3. Slightly bend at the knees.

4. Allow the dumbbells to hang down at your sides with your palms and dumbbells facing forward, as shown in the picture.

5. Make sure that your elbows stay pointed to the ground at all times during the biceps curl exercise. Do not allow them to move from that position.

6. Keep your upper body straight by sticking out your chest and keeping your shoulder blades squared off.

7. Keep your head level, and your eyes pointing straight ahead of you.

TECHNIQUE AND FORM

1. Once you are in proper postural alignment and against the wall, make sure to focus all of your attention on the biceps muscles and the exercise you are about to do. It is very easy to get distracted during exercise, but the rewards of focusing and staying focused throughout your training sessions will be well worth your efforts.

2. With the dumbbells at your sides, begin curling them up, making sure to keep your elbows pointed toward the ground.

3. Once you've reached the top position of the exercise, contract the biceps muscles as hard as you possibly can and hold that contraction for a count of 2 seconds.

4. From the top position, slowly and smoothly begin to lower the dumbbells back to the starting position.

5. As you reach the bottom of the exercise, immediately begin curling the weights up toward your shoulders again. Make sure that there is a smooth transition when switching directions from both the top position and also from the bottom position. Both scenarios must be done with no rest in between either of the direction changes, unless you are so fatigued by the end of the set that you need a few seconds of rest in order to get a couple more repetitions.

VARIATION: SUPINATION

For added stimulation of the biceps muscles, you can try a technique called supination. Instead of beginning the exercise with your palms facing forward, begin with your palms facing in toward the sides of the body. As you lift the weights, rotate your wrists until the dumbbells and palms of your hands are facing back toward you by the time you reach the top of the movement. Supination or rotation of your wrists should last the entire distance from the sides of your body up to your shoulders. In other words, don't just rotate your hands completely at the bottom position; allow them to gradually rotate during the entire distance. When you reach the top position of the exercise, your pinkies should be above your thumbs. Make sure your elbows remain pointed to the ground. Then, as you lower the weight, reverse the supination by rotating the wrists in the opposite direction, again making sure you prolong the rotation throughout the entire distance. When you finish, the palms of your hands and dumbbells should once again facing the sides of your body.

Dumbbell Curl

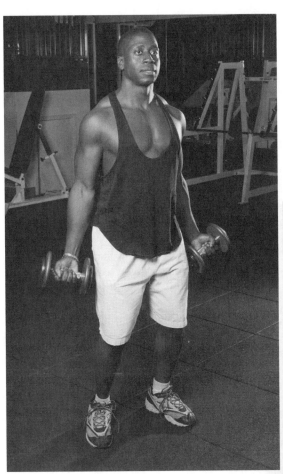

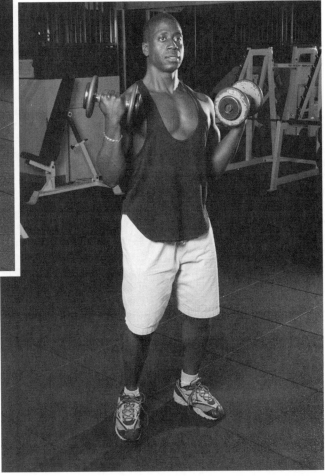

Incline Dumbbell Curl

(Using two dumbbells simultaneously)

The incline dumbbell curl is a great exercise for developing great looking biceps muscles. It was one of Arnold Schwarzenegger's favorite exercises because of the stretch that it provides at the bottom of the movement. Because the exercise requires strict form and isolation, you should start doing the exercise with a weight lighter than what you'd usually use for a regular dumbbell curl. Remember, form is everything. Make sure to avoid momentum and keep the form strict. Do not sacrifice good form for heavy weight and ego!

PROPER ALIGNMENT

1. Go to an incline bench and set the bench incline to a 45-degree angle. Due to the full stretch and range of motion of this exercise, it is designed to work the full length of the biceps with added emphasis on the outer head of the biceps muscle.

2. Pick two dumbbells with a weight that you can handle using perfect form. This exercise must be done very strictly in order to receive the desired effects.

3. Decide if you'd rather start the exercise holding the dumbbells at the sides of your body or with them resting on top of your thighs, which we prefer. Starting with the dumbbells on your thighs will give you some quality time to visualize and focus on the exercise you are about to do. This preparation can set up the proper mind-set for even greater lifting performance.

4. Lean all the way back into the bench so that your entire back is lying flat against the back pad. Stay that way for the entire exercise and do not take your back off the bench until the exercise is complete. Once you are properly positioned and ready to begin, take a firm grip on the dumbbells and allow them to hang at your sides.

5. Make sure that the palms of your hands are facing the wall in front of you for the entire exercise. No supination or hand twisting with this exercise.

6. Make sure to keep your elbows pointed directly at the floor during the entire exercise. When people usually do any type of biceps curl, they allow their elbows to drift up with the curling movement, allowing the shoulders to flex forward. When this happens, you can forget about fully stimulating the biceps muscles since the anterior shoulders become the prime movers of the weight being curled. There is only one instance that you may lift the shoulders while doing a biceps curl. That is when you have come to a point in your training where you add additional repetitions (forced reps) with the help of a spotter. Before you reach this point in your training, you must follow the earlier described form of keeping the elbows to the ground for full and proper stimulation of the biceps muscles.

TECHNIQUE AND FORM

1. Once you are in position, focus all of your attention on the exercise you are about to do and on the biceps muscle itself.

2. Begin curling the dumbbells at the same time, making sure that the elbows stay positioned towards the ground without moving upward as you curl.

3. Curl the weights up until you can no longer curl while simultaneously contracting the biceps muscles as hard as can. Hold that position for a second or two.

4. Slowly and smoothly begin to lower the dumbbells until your arms are fully elongated and back at your sides.

5. Without rest and without using any momentum, slowly and steadily begin curling the dumbbells back up toward your shoulders. If you jerk or in any way use momentum to begin curling the dumbbells, you risk serious injury to the biceps muscles. Once again, make sure that the changes of direction from the top position going into the lowering phase, and from the bottom position going into the curling phase, are always smooth and controlled.

Incline Dumbbell Curl

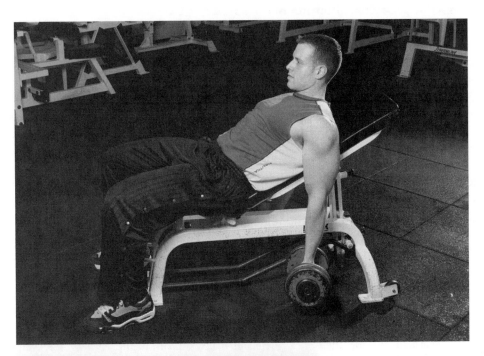

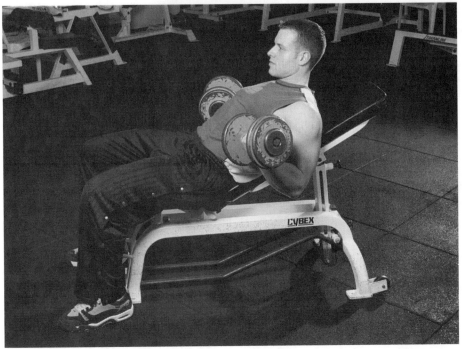

One-Arm Preacher Curl

(Using a preacher machine or inclined bench)

Larry Scott, the first Mr. Olympia, attributed his 21-inch guns to this exercise. Preacher curls develop the lower portion of the biceps muscle, helping to build balance in the biceps. For this exercise, you may use two dumbbells together or one at a time, which will help to create concentration and balance for this particular exercise. This exercise will also cause a greater contraction at the top of the movement because of the independent range of motion involved. It can be done on a preacher bench or simply on the back support of an incline bench. Because the exercise is very strict, it is important that you choose a dumbbell weight you can handle while practicing perfect form.

PROPER ALIGNMENT

1. If using a preacher machine, sit on the machine's seat and bring your chest against the pad in front of you. If using an incline bench, stand at the end of the bench so the incline portion is touching your stomach.

2. Position your feet flat on the floor and keep them there for the entire exercise.

3. Allow one arm to hang over the angled support of the preacher bench or incline bench. Support yourself with your other arm. Make sure that the back of your arm is positioned flat against the angled support and lying in a straight line. In order to comfortably keep the arm in this position, you may have to angle your body to one side making sure you are not using leveraging techniques to assist you in the curl.

4. It is important to focus all of your attention on the biceps muscles while doing the exercise instead of calling upon the assistance of other muscles to help curl the weight. Also, as you curl the weight up, make sure that you lean into the front chest support rather than lean back for cheating leverage. Make sure that the majority of the resistance is being focused on the biceps muscles throughout the exercise. When you reach the top position of the exercise, you must contract the biceps muscle as hard as you possibly can. Because you are on an angled support, the upper position of this exercise makes it very easy for you to rest the weight of the dumbbell on the bones rather than the biceps muscle sustaining the weight. You must overcome this bone support with a very hard contraction of the biceps muscle.

TECHNIQUE AND FORM

1. Once you are in position with one arm lying flat against the angled support, hold the body steady and begin curling the weight up toward your shoulder.

2. Focus all of your attention on the arm you are exercising, making sure to squeeze hard on the curling phase and resisting the weight as you come back down.

3. As you begin curling, relax the shoulder on the arm you are training as it can assist in the lift.

4. As you reach the top of this exercise, again contract the biceps muscle as hard as you can for a count of two seconds.

5. Slowly return to the starting position of the exercise.

6. As you reach the bottom position, immediately once again begin curling the weight up toward your shoulder. Once you are done with the desired amount of repetitions with that arm, switch arms and do the same amount of repetitions.

One-Arm Preacher Curl

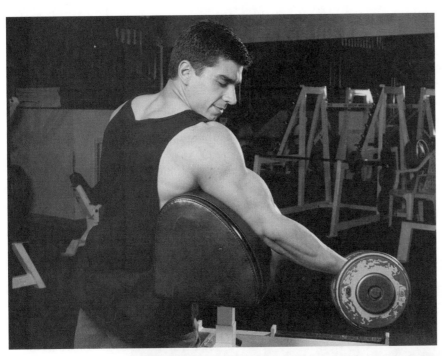

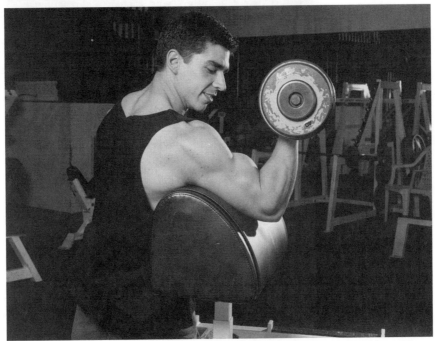

Concentration Curl

(One arm at a time)

The name concentration curl should not just be applied to this version of the biceps curl. It should be applied to every exercise we've discussed or will discuss in the book. Putting your mind into the muscle and focusing every bit of your attention on the exercise you are about to do is the surest way of reaching your fitness goals in the quickest amount of time possible. In the picture of our model demonstrating the concentration curl, look at his eyes and how they are focused on the exercise movement. His results and the results you will soon achieve are a direct result of the focus and intensity you put into every set and rep of an exercise.

PROPER ALIGNMENT

1. You can do the concentration curl either in a sitting position or while standing.

2. Whatever position you choose, bend over at the hips and take a dumbbell in one hand. The dumbbell weight should at first be light so that you can practice perfect form.

3. Sit at the edge of a bench and support your arm by resting your elbow on your thigh.

TECHNIQUE AND FORM

1. Do not curl the weight straight up to your chest. You must curl the weight with your arm angled in toward your body. This will help make certain that the exercise motion is correct, following the direction towards your shoulders rather than your chest. To start, bend over at the hips and fully extend the arm that you will be exercising while the other arm is resting on your thigh.

2. Begin curling the weight while you also begin rotating your wrist.

3. Curl the weight towards your shoulder and contract the biceps muscle as hard as you possibly can, while keeping your arm pointing at the ground.

4. Once you reach the top of the movement, hold for a 2-second count.

5. Slowly lower the dumbbell back to the starting position, resisting the weight the entire way down.

6. Without rest or momentum, once again start curling the weight towards the shoulder with great focus and concentration. Once you have completed the desired amount of repetitions, switch arms and do the same amount of repetitions.

Concentration Curl

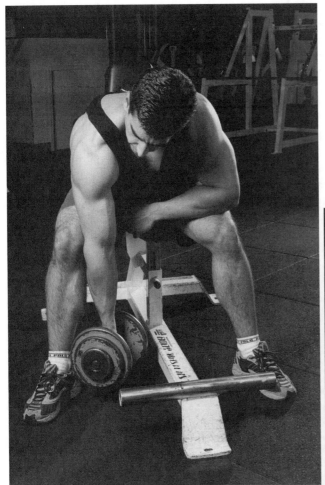

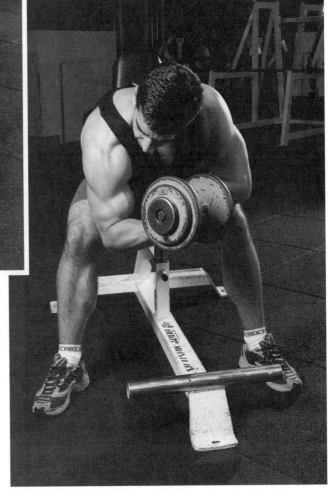

Standing E-Z Bar Curl

Do not underestimate this exercise because of its name. The E-Z bar curl is a versatile exercise that allows you to use heavy weight while being much easier on the wrists than straight bar curls. If you have a pending strain such as tennis elbow or tendonitis, we would recommend this exercise over straight bar curls. The two-curved hand positions on the bar allow you to do both close and wide-grip curls. The inner grips will enable you to develop the outer biceps, and the outer grip will enable you to develop the inner biceps.

PROPER ALIGNMENT

1. First, decide what hand position you will take on the bar. Remember what we discussed earlier about assessing your body and focusing on the unbalanced or weak body parts to create muscle balance and symmetry. Look at your biceps muscles and assess the inner and outer muscle heads. Decide if one head needs more work then the other. If you find a weakness or imbalance in one of the two muscle heads, then address that problem by simply using the hand position that will bring the smaller portion of the biceps muscle up to par with the others.

2. Hold the bar across your thighs with your palms facing away from your body.

3. Position your feet shoulder width apart and point them straight ahead. Next, bend your knees slightly.

4. Slightly contract the abdominal muscles.

5. Stand straight up and stay that way throughout the movement.

6. Stick your chest out and keep the shoulders back, which will help you maintain a straight back.

7. Keep your head level and do not move it from that position for the rest of the exercise.

TECHNIQUE AND FORM

1. With the bar across your thighs, lock your elbows to the sides of your body and begin curling the bar up towards your shoulders in an arc-like motion.

2. Keep the elbows pointing directly to the ground as you curl upward to avoid using the shoulders in the curling motion.

3. As you curl upward to the shoulders with an arc-like movement, concentrate and focus all of your attention on the biceps muscles. Feel the muscles contracting as you curl the bar upward.

4. As you reach the top of the movement with the bar close to your shoulders, contract the biceps muscles as hard as you possibly can.

5. Hold this position for a count of 1-2 seconds.

6. Slowly begin lowering the bar while making sure that the biceps endure the negative resistance on the way down to the bottom position.

7. As you reach the start position with the arms fully straightened, do not rest. Begin curling the bar once again in a smooth controlled and fluid motion without using momentum.

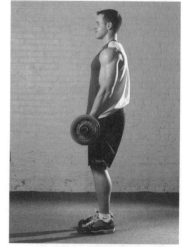

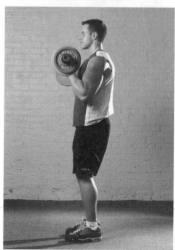

Standing E-Z Bar Curl

WIDE GRIP

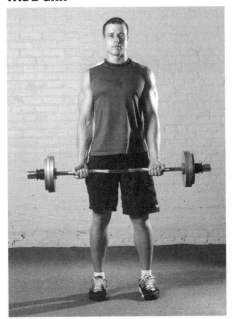
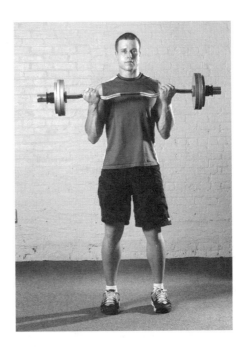

NARROW GRIP

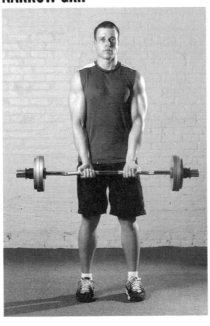
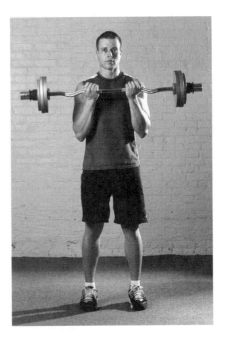

Hammer Curl

(Outer biceps and forearms)

The dumbbell hammer curl is a great exercise for building the outer head of the biceps, or brachialis muscles. It also builds the extensor muscles of the forearms. This exercise is done in the same way as standing dumbbell curls, except that you hold the dumbbells with the palms facing each other throughout the entire exercise. You can do this exercise either sitting, which will make it much stricter, or standing which will allow you to go a bit heavier. We suggest that you include both versions in your training routine.

PROPER ALIGNMENT

1. Choose two light dumbbells so that you can practice perfect form.

2. With the dumbbells in hand, begin the alignment of your body by placing your feet about shoulder width apart with the feet pointing straight ahead of you.

3. Slightly bend the knees.

4. Allow the dumbbells to hang down at your sides with your palms and dumbbells facing the sides of your body.

5. Make sure that your elbows stay pointed at the ground at all times during the biceps curl exercise.

6. Keep your upper body straight by contracting your abdominal muscles slightly, sticking out your chest and keeping your shoulder blades squared off.

7. Keep your head level, and your eyes pointing straight ahead of you.

TECHNIQUE AND FORM

1. Once you are in proper postural alignment stand against a wall. Make sure to focus all of your attention on the biceps and forearm muscles. It is very easy to get distracted during exercise, but the rewards of staying focused throughout your training sessions will be well worth your efforts.

2. Begin curling the dumbbells up with palms and dumbbells facing each other.

3. Focus on driving the thumbs to your front shoulders, concentrating on feeling the biceps and forearm muscles working.

4. Once you've reached the top position of the exercise, contract the biceps and forearm muscles as hard as you possibly can and hold that contraction for a count of 1-2 seconds.

5. From the top position, slowly and smoothly begin to lower the dumbbells back to the starting position.

6. As you reach the bottom of the exercise, the palms of your hands and dumbbells should remain facing each other and held to the sides of your body.

7. Make sure that there is a smooth transition when switching directions from both the top position going into the lowering of the dumbbells, and also from the bottom position going into the curling or raising of the dumbbells. Both scenarios must be done with no rest in between either of the direction changes, unless you are so fatigued by the end of the set that you need a few seconds rest in order to get a couple more repetitions.

Hammer Curl

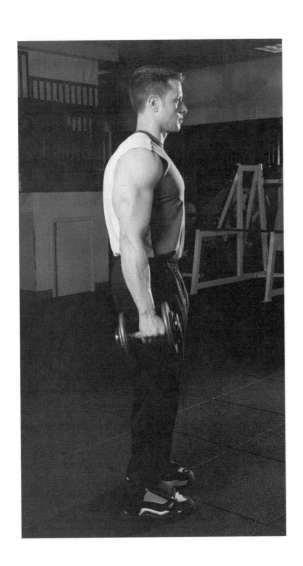

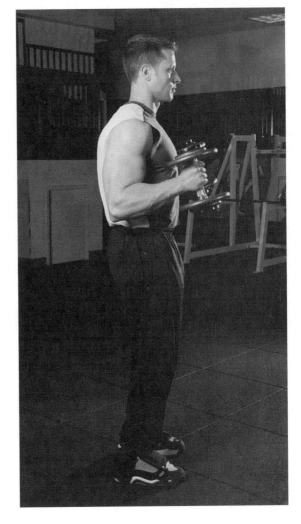

Reverse Curl

This exercise is best performed with an E-Z bar and it targets both the brachialis and the upper forearms muscles. The exercise alignment and execution is the same as that of the E-Z curls except that the hands are holding the bar with the palms facing the thighs on the outer handles of the bar for direct forearm stimulation.

PROPER ALIGNMENT

To prepare for the exercise, you will align your body similar to the way you did with the standing dumbbell biceps curl.

1. First, take your hand position by placing your hands with an overhand grip on the outer handles of the bar.

Hold the bar across your thighs with your palms facing towards your body.

2. Position your feet shoulder width apart and point them straight ahead. Next, bend your knees slightly.

3. Slightly contract the abdominal muscles.

4. Stand straight up and stay that way throughout the movement.

5. Stick your chest out and keep the shoulders back, which will help you maintain a straight back.

6. Keep your head level and do not move it from that position for the rest of the exercise.

TECHNIQUE AND FORM

1. Now in position with the bar across your thighs, lock your elbows to the sides of your body and begin curling the bar up towards your shoulders in an arc-like motion.

2. Keep the elbows pointing directly to the ground as you curl upward to avoid using the shoulders in the curling motion.

3. As you curl upward to the shoulders with an arc-like movement, concentrate and focus all of your attention on forearms and biceps muscles. Feel the muscles contracting as you curl the bar upward.

4. As you reach the top of the movement with the bar close to your shoulders, contract the biceps muscles as hard as you possibly can.

5. Hold this position for a count of 1-2 seconds.

6. Slowly begin lowering the bar while making sure that the forearms and biceps endure the negative resistance on the way back down to the bottom position.

7. As you reach the start position with the arms fully straightened, do not rest. Begin curling the bar once again in a smooth and controlled, fluid motion without using momentum.

Reverse Curl

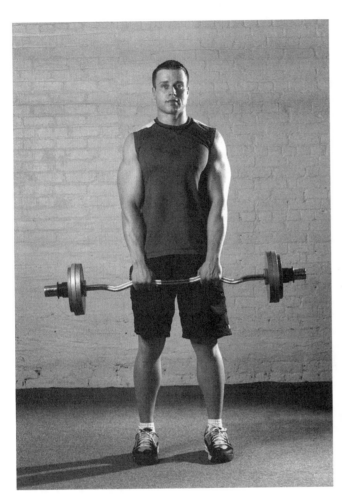

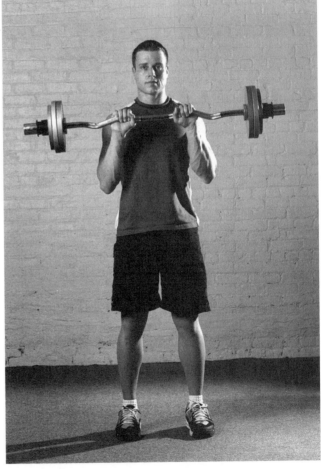

Chapter 12
Abdominals

In this section we will talk about how to exercise the most visually stunning and most sought after muscles: the abdominals. Let us recall that these exercises only firm up and build these muscles. In order to increase the visibility of the abdominal muscles, both the diet and the aerobic training have to be in order as these two are the components that burn body fat.

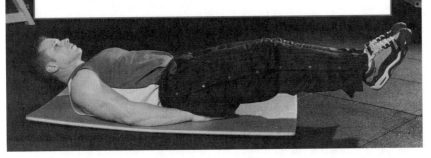

THE BODY SCULPTING BIBLE FOR MEN

Crunches

Crunches are a great exercise for the abdominal muscles. They are easier to do than the traditional sit-up (which should never be done by anyone with lower back problems) but just because they're easy doesn't mean they don't produce great results. By far, crunches are one of the best abdominal exercises for creating great looking abs as they mimic the exact function of the abdominal muscles.

PROPER ALIGNMENT

Crunches are by far one of the premier abdominal exercises for ultimate looking abs.

1. Lay down with your back flat on a carpet or mat.

2. Bend your knees and lay your feet flat on the floor.

3. Cross your hands at the chest and put a thumb on each side of your chin. This will help keep your head in a neutral position throughout the movement.

TECHNIQUE AND FORM

1. To really optimize this exercise you'll want to focus on the motion of bringing your chest plate to your pelvic area.

Our focus is to squish the stomach area between the chest and pelvis. The abdominal muscles are what will actually move your chest towards your pelvic region, so what better than to crunch them in-between the two? The reason we say this is because many trainers simply teach their clients to "crunch." Many times, instead of flexing their spines with their abdominal muscles these clients often end up using their hip flexors as the primary muscles to "crunch."

2. Begin by isometrically contracting the abdominal muscles before moving.

3. As you begin the crunch, focus on moving your chest toward your pelvis and not your head.

4. Exhale as you move up toward your knees. This will allow you to get a more forceful contraction of the abs.

5. Remember that the distance from start position to end position is not very far at all. It is not like a sit-up. Once again, your focus is not just to move but also to crunch your abs in between your chest and pelvis. Makes sense now doesn't it?

6. As you reach the top (end) position, make sure that you are contracting the abdominal muscles as hard as you possibly can. This is the most important position of the exercise.

7. Hold the contraction for a 1-2 second count.

8. Return to the bottom position and, without rest or momentum, return to the upward movement.

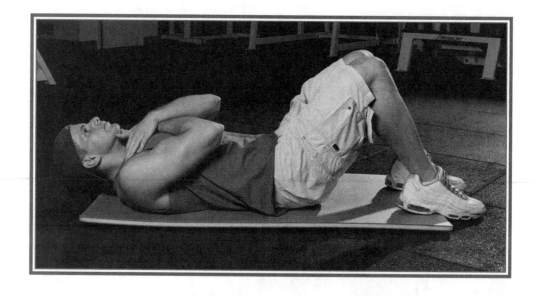

Crunches

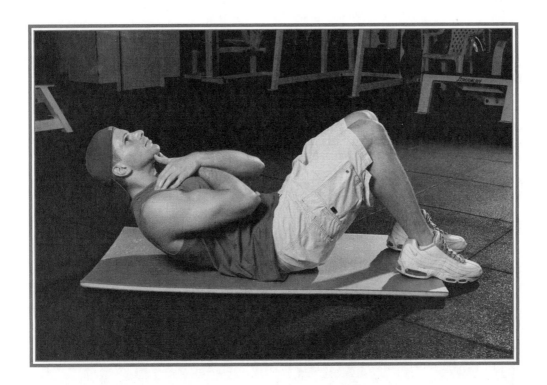

V-Up

This is a very good incorporation exercise for the upper and lower abdominal muscles. It is a variation of the crunch, but much more intense. You will simultaneously exercise the upper and lower abs. Start out easy, but try! You will soon breeze through these like a person who has an amazingly strong mid-section, because that's exactly what you'll have!

PROPER ALIGNMENT

1. Sit on the floor, making sure you are lying on a carpet or mat.

2. Put your arms by your side for support, slightly behind your torso. Your torso should be at an incline of 45 degrees between your lower back and the floor.

3. Keep the legs straight and flat on the ground.

4. Focus on keeping the head and neck in line with your chest.

5. The object is to simultaneously lift your legs and torso, thus crunching your mid-section.

TECHNIQUE AND FORM

1. Begin by isometrically contracting the abdominal muscles before moving.

2. At the same time, crunch forward by moving your torso toward your feet (as if trying to make your chest touch your legs), while you lift your legs and reverse crunch.

3. You must truly focus on the contraction of your abdominal muscles here. If you do the contraction will be very intense; a sure sign of amazing abs soon to come!

4. Hold the crunched position for a count of one second.

5. Slowly return to the start position, but do not allow your legs to touch the ground. This is a true measure of time under muscular tension and is very important if you want to obtain great results from your efforts.

6. Without rest or momentum slowly begin once again to lift your chest and legs to the middle meeting point.

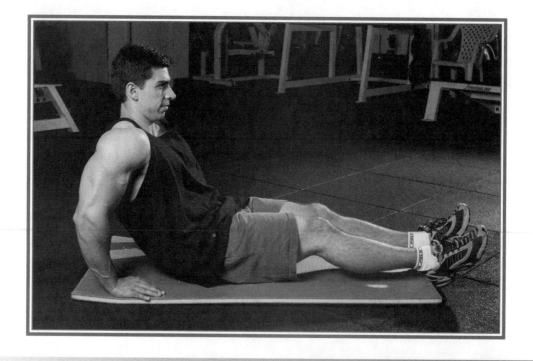

V-Up

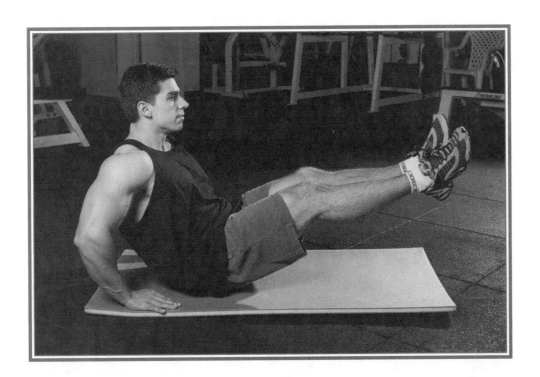

Leg Raise

Leg raises are a great lower abdominal exercise. It is not enough though to simply lift the legs off of the floor. Doing so can hurt the lower back and will do nothing to improve your lower abdominal muscles. You must focus and feel the abdominal muscles actually working while you raise your legs up. When you are ready for the next step, WATCH OUT! The advanced version of the leg raise will not only blow your mind, but will blast your abdominal results into the stratosphere!

PROPER ALIGNMENT

1. Lay flat on the floor with your legs straight and flat on the floor as well.

2. Put your hands face down underneath your buttocks, with fingertips facing each other. Your ring finger and pinky finger will most likely sit between the insertion point of your buttocks and hamstrings. This is a preventative measure against lower back injury.

3. You will also put a very slight bend in the knees for the same reason.

TECHNIQUE AND FORM

1. Begin by lifting your legs about 5 inches off the ground and holding. This is for preparation.

2. Lift your legs straight up until they are perpendicular to the ground.

3. Make sure you are focused on the abdominal muscles working while you move the legs up.

4. When you reach the vertical point, squeeze the abs as hard as you can and hold momentarily.

5. Slowly return the legs to the bottom position but remember to stop 5 inches from the floor. From here you will once again lift the legs up.

ADVANCED VERSION

This time when your legs reach the point the perpendicular position, holding the vertical position, lift your buttocks off of your hands and reach your feet into the air as if you are trying to put footprints on the ceiling. This little movement will greatly enhance the stimulation of the lower abdominal section. It is like doing an instant superset and is sure to be one of your favorites.

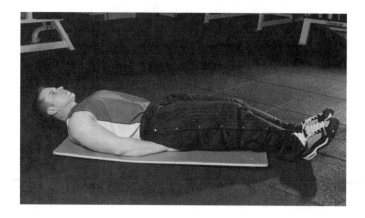

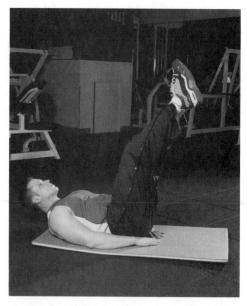

Leg Raise

ADVANCED

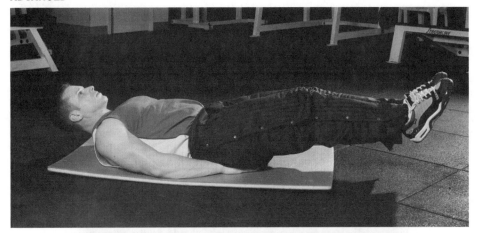

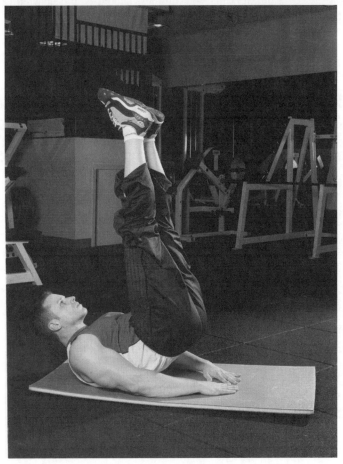

Trunk Curl and Crunch

This is yet another incorporation exercise, simultaneously working the upper and lower abs. You should find this easier than the V-Ups but just as effective. The object is to bring the knees to the chest and chest to the knees at the same time.

PROPER ALIGNMENT

1. Lay flat on your back with knees bent, but lower legs and feet suspended (The correct thigh and lower leg position should look like the number 7).

2. As you did with the crunch curl, cross your hands across your chest with your thumbs touching each side of your chin.

3. Once again, the object will be to simultaneously crunch your chest to your knees and your knees to your chest. The elbows will meet with the knees as an indicator of one full rep.

TECHNIQUE AND FORM

1. Cross your hands over your chest and bring the thighs and feet away from your body in front of you. This will provide a full range of motion for this exercise.

2. Isometrically contract the abdominal muscles before moving.

3. At the same time, crunch your chest to your knees and bring your knees to your chest. Your back should come off the ground while your buttocks should also slightly lift off the ground.

4. By touching your elbows to the knees and vice-versa you will know you have done one full rep. It is at this point that you should squeeze the abdominal muscles as hard as you possibly can. Do not cheat by failing to bring your thighs away from your body in front of you. With each rep, reach out with your feet and allow the lower abs to bring them back in for the knee-elbow touch. At the same time, do not fail to effectively crunch your upper body from the bottom of the floor up to the elbow-knee touch.

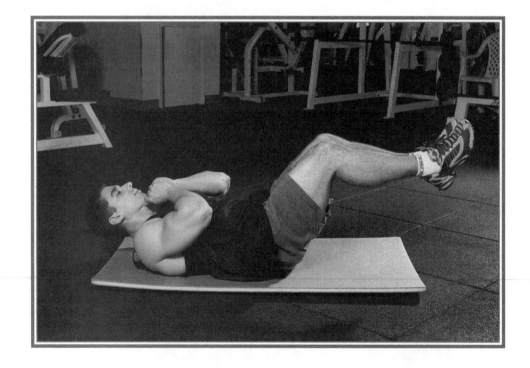

Trunk Curl and Crunch

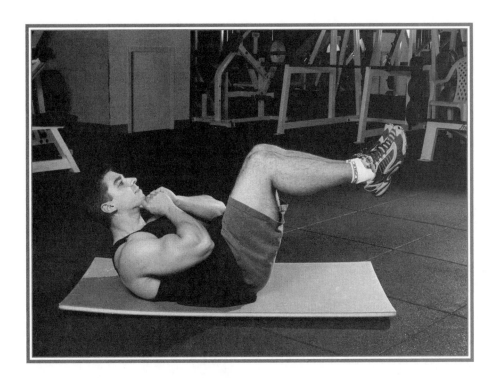

Knee-Ins

This is another great variation exercise for developing the lower abdominal muscles.

It is more convenient than some of the other lower abdominal exercises and just as effective. This exercise also gives you the ability to really squeeze the lower abs when the knees are brought in towards your chest. For a change of pace, vary your speed from one workout to the next. The next time you do this or any of the exercises we recommend, move slowly while exercising. Deliberately squeeze the abdominal muscles at the peak contraction position. Then the next time you train your abdominal muscles again, go a little quicker. This variation in the speed of your movements will help to keep your body from hitting a plateau, while keeping you motivated by changing the pace of your movements.

PROPER ALIGNMENT

1. Sit on the floor (or on the edge of a chair or exercise bench) with your legs extended in front of you.

2. Your hands should be holding on to the sides of the bench or to the floor for support.

TECHNIQUE AND FORM

1. Keeping your knees together, pull them in towards your chest until you can go no farther.

2. Keeping the tension on your lower abdominal muscles, return to the start position.

3. Repeat the movement until you have completed your set.

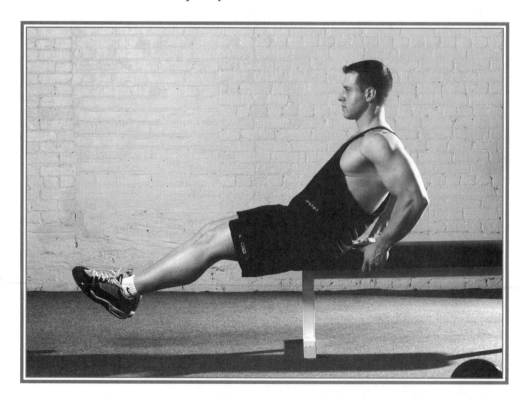

Knee-Ins

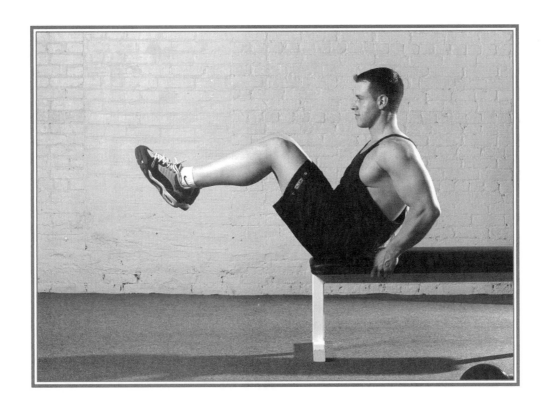

FINAL POINTERS ON EXERCISE FORM

Remember that without knowing how to perform an exercise correctly, no matter how good your routine is you will not get the fast results that you want and deserve.

Also keep in mind that before starting any exercise, you should think about or visualize yourself doing the movement. This helps prepare you better for the exercise. When you begin the exercise, mentally focus on the muscle you are trying to stimulate. Use the Zone-Tone technique.

Remember how powerful the mind is and what it can do! By focusing your attention and "putting your mind in the muscle" you will double the intensity of muscle stimulation and therefore double your results. This is opposed to simply allowing any available muscle in the body to move the weight merely by going through the motions. You must learn to be connected as one with the muscle, observant of the connection every moment during the movement. Picture your muscle as toned and as lean as you want it to be. It's really much easier than you would expect to master the mind-to-muscle connection and you'll soon see remarkable results from your newfound knowledge and dedication.

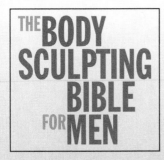

THE **BODY**
SCULPTING
BIBLE
FOR **MEN**

Part 4
Workout Charts

Chapter 13
Workout Charts

13

THE BREAK-IN PROGRAM

In this program you will train with weights 4 days a week and perform aerobic activity 2 days a week. In this book we use Sundays as your off days. You may do Day 1 on Mondays and Thursdays, Day 2 on Tuesdays and Fridays and Day 3 on Wednesdays and Saturdays.

This program is designed to be performed in the comfort of your home with minimum equipment, namely a pair of dumbbells or a pair of dumbbells with an adjustable bench. As you get stronger you may wish to purchase a pair of secure adjustable dumbbells such as Powerblocks.

You will notice that we present two Break-In Routines. The first routine is designed on the assumption that the only equipment available is a pair of dumbbells. The second routine is based on the assumption that you also have access to an adjustable exercise bench with a leg curl/leg extension attachment. Choose the routine that you can do with the equipment you have available.

HOW TO PROGRESS WITH BREAK-IN ROUTINES 1 & 2

For the first six weeks, follow the routine exactly as it is laid out. The reason for this is that if you have never worked out before, it will take your body approximately six weeks to adjust and get used to the movements, while making it most efficient for recruiting muscle fibers. It will also give your cardiovascular system a chance to start getting back into shape. By the end of the six weeks, you should have lost a significant amount of weight and you should start seeing more muscle tone and definition in your body. You should also be able to reach your target heart rate by the end of this period.

After week 6, add one more set to all of the exercises. You will now be performing three sets instead of two. Increase the weights and perform fewer repetitions (13-15; except for abs and calves where the repetition range stays the same). Also, increase your aerobic activity to 20 minutes. Follow this workout for the next 4 weeks.

After week 10, you are ready to go up to 4 sets per exercise and 30 minutes of cardio. Increase the weights and perform fewer repetitions (10-12; except for abs and calves where the repetition range stays the same). Follow this workout for three more weeks and then you should not only look dramatically different, but you are also in perfect shape to start the 14-Day Body Sculpting Workout

THE 14-DAY BODY SCULPTING WORKOUT

In this program you will train with weights 4 days a week and perform aerobic activity 2 days a week. Sundays are your off days. You may do Day 1 on Mondays and Thursdays, Day 2 on Tuesdays and Fridays and Day 3 on Wednesdays and Saturdays.

This program is designed to be performed in the comfort of your home with minimum equipment, namely a pair of dumbbells or a pair of dumbbells with an adjustable bench. As you get stronger you may wish to purchase a pair of secure adjustable dumbbells such as Powerblocks.

You will notice that we present two 14-Day Body Sculpting Workouts. The first routine is designed on the assumption that the only equipment available is a pair of dumbbells. The second routine is based on the assumption that you also have access to an adjustable exercise bench with a leg curl/leg extension attachment. Choose the routine that you can do with the equipment that you have available.

THE ADVANCED 14-DAY BODY SCULPTING WORKOUT

In this program you will train with weights 6 days a week and perform aerobic activity 6 days a week. Sundays are your off days. You may do Day 1 on Mondays and Thursdays, Day 2 on Tuesdays and Fridays and Day 3 on Wednesdays and Saturdays.

This program is designed to be performed at either a commercial gym or a very well equipped home gym. The reason for this is that we will be using a variety of exercises and training different angles and areas of the muscles in order to stimulate all muscle fibers.

Cardio and abs are to be performed on a daily basis preferably first thing in the morning on an empty stomach. The weight training workouts are to be performed in the afternoon or at any other convenient time.

THE 14-DAY BODY SCULPTING MASS WORKOUT

This program was created for those people with faster metabolisms—and consequently, low body fat—who are interested only in gaining muscle. We created the program with the assumption that you will be working out at a well-equipped gym. If you are working out at home, just substitute exercises that you can do with your equipment for those designed for the gym. However, be aware that to add serious muscle you will have to lift some heavy weights, which means that you need sturdy, high-quality equipment. At this point, you should have already completed the Break-In Routines described earlier. If you are a complete beginner, start with the Break-In Routines. Once you have completed them, you can graduate to this level.

You will notice that every two weeks the exercises change along with the set, rep and rest schemes to provide a fresh shock to the body. If you work out at a gym, once you have completed this routine, feel free to add other exercises, such leg press hack squats for the leg routines. As long as the exercises are basic (using mostly free weights), there is no problem with substituting them for other exercises.

Break-In Routine #1

DAY 1

Modified Compound Superset # 1
Back—Dumbbell Rows (one arm)   *138*
Reps: 15-20   Sets: 2
Rest: 90 seconds
Chest—Push-ups (against the wall
if unable to perform on the floor)   *172*
Reps: 15-20   Sets: 2
Rest: 90 seconds

Modified Compound Superset # 2
Back—Dumbbell Rows (two arms)   *138*
Reps: 15-20   Sets: 2
Rest: 90 seconds
Chest —Flat Dumbbell Flys   *164*
(performed on the floor if you don't
have access to an exercise bench)
Reps: 15-20   Sets: 2
Rest: 90 seconds

Modified Compound Superset # 3
Biceps—Dumbbell Curls   *212*
Reps: 15-20   Sets: 2
Rest: 90 seconds
Triceps—Lying Dumbbell
Extensions   *194*
Reps: 15-20   Sets: 2
Rest: 90 seconds

Modified Compound Superset # 4
Biceps—Hammer Curls   *222*
Reps: 15-20   Sets: 2
Rest: 90 seconds
Triceps—Overhead Dumbbell
Extensions   *192*
Reps: 15-20   Sets: 2
Rest: 90 seconds

DAY 2

Modified Compound Superset # 1
Thighs—Dumbbell Squats   *104*
Reps: 15-20   Sets: 2
Rest: 90 seconds
Hamstrings—Dumbbell Lunges   *108*
Reps: 15-20   Sets: 2
Rest: 90 seconds

Modified Compound Superset # 2
Thighs—Ballet Squats   *106*
Reps: 15-20   Sets: 2
Rest: 90 seconds
Hamstrings—Stiff-legged Deadlifts   *120*
Reps: 15-20   Sets: 2
Rest: 90 seconds

Modified Compound Superset # 3
Calves—Standing Calf Raises   *124*
(one leg)
Reps: 15-25   Sets: 2
Rest: 90 seconds
Shoulders—Dumbbell Shoulder
Press   *178*
Reps: 15-20   Sets: 2
Rest: 90 seconds

Modified Compound Superset # 4
Calves—Standing Calf Raises   *124*
(two legs using dumbbells)
Reps: 15-25   Sets: 2
Rest: 90 seconds
Shoulders—Bent-Over Lateral
Raises   *186*
Reps: 15-20   Sets: 2
Rest: 90 seconds

Break-In Routine #1

DAY 3

Modified Compound Superset # 1

Lower Abs—*Leg Raises*   232
Reps: 15-25   Sets: 2
Rest: 90 seconds

Upper Abs—*Crunches*   228
Reps: 15-25   Sets: 2
Rest: 90 seconds

AEROBIC ACTIVITY

10 minutes of fast walking, stationary bike, or any other type of aerobic activity that you like. Don't be concerned at this stage with reaching the target heart rate. Just concentrate on performing the activity at a comfortable but steady pace.

NOTES:

Repetitions

You will note that the repetition ranges are higher than what we normally recommend, which means using lighter weights, for the following reasons.

To start getting the joints and muscles accustomed to weight training exercise while preventing injuries.
To start creating neural pathways (links) between the brain and the muscles so that you start gaining better control and feel of the muscles in your body.

Abs

If you cannot perform the desired amount of repetitions for abdominal exercises, just do as many as you can and as your strength allows, increase the number of reps.

Pushups

Depending on your bodyweight you may find this exercise difficult to do in the traditional manner. If this is the case, then start by performing them standing against the wall (stand 1.5-2 ft in front of the wall, extend your arms and perform the exercise) as in this manner you will not be lifting your full bodyweight. As you become stronger, you may perform them on the floor in the "halfway" position. This is when you will kneel down and perform the push-up the same way you would regularly with the exception of not keeping your legs straight Once you master that position, you will be able to perform the traditional pushup.

Break-In Routine #2

SPECIAL INSTRUCTIONS FOR WEEKS 1 & 2

Use modified compound supersets. Perform Modified Compound Supersets by performing the first exercise, resting for the prescribed rest period, performing the second exercise, resting the prescribed rest period and going back to the first exercise. Continue in this manner until you have performed all of the prescribed number of sets. Then continue with the next modified compound superset.

DAY 1

Modified Compound Superset # 1
Back—Dumbbell Rows   138
(one arm, alternate with two-arm rows
on the next workout)
Reps: 15-20   Sets: 2
Rest: 90 seconds
Chest—Incline Dumbbell Press   160
Reps: 15-20   Sets: 2
Rest: 90 seconds

Modified Compound Superset # 2
Back—Dumbbell Pullovers   150
Reps: 15-20   Sets: 2
Rest: 90 seconds
Chest—Incline Dumbbell Flys   166
(alternate with Push-ups on the next
workout, 172)
Reps: 15-20   Sets: 2
Rest: 90 seconds

Modified Compound Superset # 3
Biceps—Dumbbell Curls   212
Reps: 15-20   Sets: 2
Rest: 90 seconds
Triceps—Lying Dumbbell Extensions 194
Reps: 15-20   Sets: 2
Rest: 90 seconds

Modified Compound Superset # 4
Biceps—Concentration Curls   218
(alternate with Hammer Curls, 222)
Reps: 15-20   Sets: 2
Rest: 90 seconds
Triceps—Triceps Kickbacks   208
(alternate with Overhead Dumbbell
Extensions, 192)
Reps: 15-20   Sets: 2
Rest: 90 seconds

DAY 2

Modified Compound Superset # 1
Thighs—Dumbbell Squats   104
(alternate with Ballet Squats, 106)
Reps: 15-20   Sets: 2
Rest: 90 seconds
Hamstrings—Leg Curls   116
(alternate with Dumbbell Lunges, 108)
Reps: 15-20   Sets: 2
Rest: 90 seconds

Modified Compound Superset # 2
Thighs—Ballet Squats   106
(alternate with Leg Extensions, 112)
Reps: 15-20   Sets: 2
Rest: 90 seconds
Hamstrings—Stiff-legged Deadlifts 120
(Alternate with Leg Curls, 114)
Reps: 15-20   Sets: 2
Rest: 90 seconds

Modified Compound Superset # 3
Calves—Standing Calf Raises   124
(one leg)
Reps: 15-25   Sets: 2
Rest: 90 seconds
Shoulders—Dumbbell Shoulder   178
Press
(alternate with Upright Rows, 184)
Reps: 15-20   Sets: 2
Rest: 90 seconds

Modified Compound Superset # 4
Calves—Standing Calf Raises   124
(two legs)
Reps: 15-25   Sets: 2
Rest: 90 seconds
Shoulders—Bent-Over Lateral
Raises   186
Reps: 15-20   Sets: 2
Rest: 90 seconds

Break-In Routine #2

DAY 3

Modified Compound Superset # 1
Lower Abs—*Leg Raises*   232
Reps: 15-25   Sets: 2
Rest: 90 seconds

Upper Abs—*Crunches*   228
Reps: 15-25   Sets: 2
Rest: 90 seconds

AEROBIC ACTIVITY

10 minutes of fast walking, stationary bike, or any other type of aerobic activity that you like. Don't be concerned at this stage with reaching the target heart rate. Just concentrate on performing the activity at a comfortable but steady pace.

NOTES:

Repetitions
You will note that the repetition ranges are higher than what we normally recommend, which means using lighter weights, for the following reasons:

In order to start getting the joints and muscles accustomed to weight training exercise while preventing injuries.
In order to start creating neural pathways between the brain and muscles so you start gaining better control and feel of the muscles in your body.

Abs
If you cannot perform the desired amount of repetitions for abdominal exercises, just do as many as you can. As your strength allows, increase the number of reps.

Push-ups
Depending on your bodyweight you may find this exercise difficult to do in the traditional way. If this is the case, start by performing them standing against the wall (stand 1.5-2 ft in front of the wall, extend your arms and perform the exercise) as in this manner you will not be lifting your full bodyweight. As you become stronger, you may perform them on the floor in the "halfway" position. This is when you will kneel down and perform the push-up the same way you would regularly with the exception of not keeping your legs straight. Once you master that position, you will be able to perform the traditional pushup.

ALTERNATE EXERCISES
Alternate exercises are added as a means to introduce variety into the weight-training program. Variety is good as it prevents the body from getting used to the exercise routine, helping to avoid boredom. It also helps to intensify your workouts by providing additional angles of movement for diversified muscular stimulation.

These alternate exercises are to be performed in the second workout of the week. For instance, if you did Ballet Squats on Tuesday, then do Leg Extensions instead on Friday.

14-Day Body Sculpting Workout #1

SPECIAL INSTRUCTIONS FOR WEEKS 1 & 2

Use modified compound supersets. Perform modified compound supersets by performing the first exercise, resting for the prescribed rest period, performing the second exercise, resting the prescribed rest period and going back to the first exercise. Continue in this manner until you have performed all of the prescribed number of sets. Then continue with the next modified compound superset.

Day 1

Modified Compound Superset # 1
Back—*Dumbbell Rows (one arm)*   138
Reps: 12-15   Sets: 2
Rest: 90 seconds
Chest—*Push-ups*   172
(against the wall if unable to perform on the floor)
Reps: 12-15   Sets: 2
Rest: 90 seconds

Modified Compound Superset # 2
Back —*Dumbbell Rows (two arms)*   138
Reps: 12-15   Sets: 2
Rest: 90 seconds
Chest—*Flat Dumbbell Flys*   164
(performed on the floor if you don't have access to an exercise bench)
Reps: 12-15   Sets: 2
Rest: 90 seconds

Modified Compound Superset # 3
Biceps-*Dumbbell Curls*   212
Reps: 12-15   Sets: 2
Rest: 90 seconds
Triceps—*Lying Dumbbell Extensions* 194
Reps: 12-15   Sets: 2
Rest: 90 seconds

Modified Compound Superset # 4
Biceps—*Hammer Curls*   222
Reps: 12-15   Sets: 2
Rest: 90 seconds
Triceps—*Overhead Dumbbell Extensions*   192
Reps: 12-15   Sets: 2
Rest: 90 seconds

DAY 2

Modified Compound Superset # 1
Thighs—*Dumbbell Squats*   104
(alternate with Ballet Squats, 106)
Reps: 12-15   Sets: 2
Rest: 90 seconds
Hamstrings—*Dumbbell Lunges*   108
Reps: 12-15   Sets: 2
Rest: 90 seconds

Modified Compound Superset # 2
Thighs—*Ballet Squats*   106
Reps: 12-15   Sets: 2
Rest: 90 seconds
Hamstrings—*Stiff-legged Deadlifts* 114
Reps: 12-15   Sets: 2
Rest: 90 seconds

Modified Compound Superset # 3
Calves—*Standing Calf Raises*   124
(one leg)
Reps: 12-15   Sets: 2
Rest: 90 seconds
Shoulders—*Dumbbell Shoulder Press*   178
Reps: 12-15   Sets: 2
Rest: 90 seconds

Modified Compound Superset # 4
Calves—*Standing Calf Raises*   124
(two legs)
Reps: 12-15   Sets: 2
Rest: 90 seconds
Shoulders—*Bent-Over Lateral Raises*   186
Reps: 12-15   Sets: 2
Rest: 90 second

DAY 3

Modified Compound Superset # 1

Lower Abs—*Leg Raises*   *232*
Reps: 15-25   Sets: 2
Rest: 90 seconds
Upper Abs—*Crunches*   *228*
Reps: 15-25   Sets: 2
Rest: 90 seconds

AEROBIC ACTIVITY

20 minutes of fast walking, stationary bike, or any other
type of aerobic activity that you like at the target heart rate.

14-Day Body Sculpting Workout #1

SPECIAL INSTRUCTIONS FOR WEEKS 3 & 4

Use supersets. Perform supersets by pairing exercises with no rest period in between. Only rest after the two exercises have been performed consecutively. Repeat for the prescribed number of sets and then move on to the next pair of exercises.

DAY 1

Superset # 1
Back—*Dumbbell Rows (one arm)*   *138*
Reps: 10-12   Sets: 3
Rest: No Rest
Chest—*Push-ups*   *172*
(against the wall if unable to perform on the floor)
Reps: 10-12   Sets: 3
Rest: 60 seconds

Superset # 2
Back—*Dumbbell Rows (two arms)*   *138*
Reps: 10-12   Sets: 3
Rest: No Rest
Chest—*Flat Dumbbell Flys*   *164*
(performed on the floor if you don't have access to an exercise bench)
Reps: 10-12   Sets: 3
Rest: 60 seconds

Superset # 3
Biceps—*Dumbbell Curls*   *212*
Reps: 10-12   Sets: 3
Rest: No Rest
Triceps—*Lying Dumbbell Extensions* *194*
Reps: 10-12   Sets: 3
Rest: 60 seconds

Superset # 4
Biceps—*Hammer Curls*   *222*
Reps: 10-12   Sets: 3
Rest: No Rest
Triceps—*Overhead Dumbbell Extensions*   *192*
Reps: 10-12   Sets: 3
Rest: 60 seconds

DAY 2

Superset # 1
Thighs—*Dumbbell Squats*   *104*
Reps: 10-12   Sets: 3
Rest: No Rest
Hamstrings—*Dumbbell Lunges*   *108*
Reps: 10-12   Sets: 3
Rest: 60 seconds

Superset # 2
Thighs—*Ballet Squats*   *106*
Reps: 10-12   Sets: 3
Rest: No Rest
Hamstrings—*Stiff-legged Deadlifts* *120*
Reps: 10-12   Sets: 3
Rest: 60 seconds

Superset # 3
Calves—*Standing Calf Raises*   *124*
(one leg)
Reps: 12-15   Sets: 3
Rest: No Rest
Shoulders—*Dumbbell Shoulder Press*   *178*
Reps: 10-12   Sets: 3
Rest: 60 seconds

Superset # 4
Calves—*Standing Calf Raises*   *124*
(two legs)
Reps: 12-15   Sets: 3
Rest: No Rest
Shoulders—*Bent-Over Lateral Raises*   *186*
Reps: 10-12   Sets: 3
Rest: 60 seconds

Weeks 3 & 4

DAY 3

Superset # 1

Lower Abs—*Leg Raises*   232
Reps: 15-25   Sets: 3
Rest: No Rest

Upper Abs—*Crunches*   228
Reps: 15-25   Sets: 3
Rest: 90 seconds

AEROBIC ACTIVITY

30 minutes of fast walking, stationary bike, or any other type of aerobic activity that you like at your target heart rate.

14-Day Body Sculpting Workout #1

SPECIAL INSTRUCTIONS FOR WEEKS 5 & 6

Use giant sets. Perform giant sets by performing four exercises with no rest period in between. Only rest after the four exercises have been performed consecutively. Repeat for the prescribed number of sets and then move on to the second group of exercises.

DAY 1

Giant set # 1

Back—*Dumbbell Rows (one arm)*   138
Reps: 8-10   Sets: 4
Rest: No rest

Chest—*Push-ups*   172
(against the wall if unable to perform on the floor)
Reps: 8-10   Sets: 4
Rest: No rest

Back—*Dumbbell Rows (two arms)*   138
Reps: 8-10   Sets: 4
Rest: No rest

Chest—*Flat Dumbbell Flys*   164
(performed on the floor if you don't have access to an exercise bench)
Reps: 8-10   Sets: 4
Rest: 60 seconds

Giant set # 2

Biceps—*Dumbbell Curls*   212
Reps: 8-10   Sets: 4
Rest: No rest

Triceps—*Lying Dumbbell Extensions* 194
Reps: 8-10   Sets: 4
Rest: No rest

Biceps—*Hammer Curls*   222
Reps: 8-10   Sets: 4
Rest: No rest

Triceps-*Overhead Dumbbell Extensions*   192
Reps: 8-10   Sets: 4
Rest: 60 seconds

Day 2

Giant set # 1

Thighs—*Dumbbell Squats*   104
Reps: 8-10   Sets: 4
Rest: No rest

Hamstrings—*Dumbbell Lunges*   108
Reps: 8-10   Sets: 4
Rest: No rest

Thighs—*Ballet Squats*   106
Reps: 8-10   Sets: 4
Rest: No rest

Hamstrings—*Stiff-legged Deadlifts* 120
Reps: 8-10   Sets: 4
Rest: 60 seconds

Giant set # 2

Calves—*Standing Calf Raises (one leg)*   124
Reps: 15-25   Sets: 4
Rest: No rest

Shoulders—*Dumbbell Shoulder Press*   178
Reps: 15-25   Sets: 4
Rest: No rest

Calves—*Standing Calf Raises (two legs)*   124
Reps: 15-25   Sets: 4
Rest: No rest

Shoulders—*Bent-Over Lateral Raises*   186
Reps: 15-25   Sets: 4
Rest: 60 seconds

Weeks 5 & 6

DAY 3

Giant set # 1

Lower Abs—*Leg Raises*   232
Reps: 15-25   Sets: 4
Rest: No Rest

Upper Abs—*Crunches*   228
Reps: 15-25   Sets: 4
Rest: No Rest

(**Note:** Continue until all four sets of each exercise have
been done. Don't worry if you are not able to perform all of
the recommended reps the first few times that you perform
this abdominal workout. As you get used to this rigorous
workout, your body will adapt and get stronger).

Aerobic Activity
40 minutes of fast walking, stationary bike, or any
other type of aerobic activity that you like at your
target heart rate.

14-Day Body Sculpting Workout #2

SPECIAL INSTRUCTIONS FOR WEEKS 1 & 2

Use modified compound supersets. Perform modified compound supersets by performing the first exercise, resting for the prescribed rest period, performing the second exercise, resting the prescribed rest period and going back to the first exercise. Continue in this manner until you have performed all of the prescribed number of sets. Then continue with the next modified compound superset.

Day 1

Modified Compound Superset # 1
Back—Dumbbell Rows   138
(one arm, alternate with two arms
on the next workout)
Reps: 12-15   Sets: 2
Rest: 90 seconds
Chest—Incline Dumbbell Press   160
Reps: 12-15   Sets: 2
Rest: 90 seconds

Modified Compound Superset # 2
Back—Dumbbell Pullovers   150
Reps: 12-15   Sets: 2
Rest: 90 seconds
Chest—Incline Dumbbell Flys   166
(alternate with Push-ups)
Reps: 12-15   Sets: 2
Rest: 90 seconds

Modified Compound Superset # 3
Biceps—Dumbbell Curls   212
Reps: 12-15   Sets: 2
Rest: 90 seconds
Triceps—Lying Dumbbell Extensions 194
Reps: 12-15   Sets: 2
Rest: 90 seconds

Modified Compound Superset # 4
Biceps—Concentration Curls   218
(alternate with Hammer Curls, 222)
Reps: 12-15   Sets: 2
Rest: 90 seconds
Triceps—Triceps Kickbacks   208
(alternate with Overhead Dumbbell
Extensions, 192)
Reps: 12-15   Sets: 2
Rest: 90 seconds

Day 2

Modified Compound Superset # 1
Thighs—Dumbbell Squats   104
(alternate with Ballet Squats, 106)
Reps: 12-15   Sets: 2
Rest: 90 seconds
Hamstrings—Lying Leg Curls   114
(alternate with Dumbbell Lunges, 108)
Reps: 12-15   Sets: 2
Rest: 90 seconds

Modified Compound Superset # 2
Thighs—Ballet Squats   106
(alternate with Leg Extensions, 112)
Reps: 12-15   Sets: 2
Rest: 90 seconds
Hamstrings—Stiff-legged Deadlifts 120
(alternate with Standing Leg Curls, 118)
Reps: 12-15   Sets: 2
Rest: 90 seconds

Modified Compound Superset # 3
Calves—Standing Calf Raises   124
(one leg)
Reps: 12-15   Sets: 2
Rest: 90 seconds
Shoulders—Dumbbell Shoulder
Press   178
(Alternate with Upright Rows, 184)
Reps: 12-15   Sets: 2
Rest: 90 seconds

Modified Compound Superset # 4
Calves—Standing Calf Raises   124
(two legs)
Reps: 12-15   Sets: 2
Rest: 90 seconds
Shoulders—Bent-Over Lateral
Raises   186
Reps: 12-15   Sets: 2
Rest: 90 seconds

DAY 3

Modified Compound Superset # 1

Lower Abs—*Leg Raises*   232
Reps: 15-25   Sets: 2
Rest: 90 seconds
Upper Abs—*Crunches*   228
Reps: 15-25   Sets: 2
Rest: 90 seconds

AEROBIC ACTIVITY

20 minutes of fast walking, stationary bike, or any
other type of aerobic activity that you like at your
target heart rate.

14-Day Body Sculpting Workout #2

> ## SPECIAL INSTRUCTIONS FOR WEEKS 3 & 4
>
> Use supersets. Perform supersets by pairing exercises with no rest period in between. Only rest after the two exercises have been performed consecutively. Repeat for the prescribed number of sets and then move on to the next pair of exercises.

DAY 1

Superset # 1
Back—Dumbbell Rows   138
(one arm, alternate with two arms
on the next workout)
Reps: 10-12   Sets: 3
Rest: No Rest
Chest—Incline Dumbbell Press   160
Reps: 10-12   Sets: 3
Rest: 60 seconds

Superset # 2
Back—Dumbbell Pullovers   150
Reps: 10-12   Sets: 3
Rest: No Rest
Chest—Incline Dumbbell Flys   166
(alternate with Push-ups, 172)
Reps: 10-12   Sets: 3
Rest: 60 seconds

Superset # 3
Biceps—Dumbbell Curls   212
Reps: 10-12   Sets: 3
Rest: No Rest
Triceps—Lying Dumbbell Extensions 194
Reps: 10-12   Sets: 3
Rest: 60 seconds

Superset # 4
Biceps—Concentration Curls   218
(alternate with Hammer Curls, 222)
Reps: 10-12   Sets: 3
Rest: No Rest
Triceps—Triceps Kickbacks   208
(alternate with Overhead Dumbbell
Extensions, 192)
Reps: 10-12   Sets: 3
Rest: 60 seconds

DAY 2

Superset # 1
Thighs—Dumbbell Squats   104
(alternate with Ballet Squats, 106)
Reps: 10-12   Sets: 3
Rest: No Rest
Hamstrings—Lying Leg Curls   114
(alternate with Dumbbell Lunges, 108)
Reps: 10-12   Sets: 3
Superset # 2
Thighs—Ballet Squats   106
(alternate with Leg Extensions, 112)
Reps: 10-12   Sets: 3
Rest: No Rest
Hamstrings—Stiff-legged Deadlifts   120
(alternate with Standing Leg Curls, 118)
Reps: 10-12   Sets: 3
Rest: 60 seconds

Superset # 3
Calves—Standing Calf Raises   124
(one leg)
Reps: 12-15   Sets: 3
Rest: No Rest
Shoulders—Dumbbell Shoulder
Press   178
(alternate with Upright Rows, 184)
Reps: 10-12   Sets: 3
Rest: 60 seconds

Superset # 4
Calves—Standing Calf Raises   124
(two legs)
Reps: 12-15   Sets: 3
Rest: No Rest
Shoulders—Bent-Over Lateral
Raises   186
Reps: 10-12   Sets: 3
Rest: 60 seconds

DAY 3

Superset # 1
Lower Abs*—Leg Raises*   *232*
Reps: 15-25   Sets: 3
Rest: No Rest
Upper Abs*—Crunches*   *228*
Reps: 15-25   Sets: 3
Rest: 90 seconds

AEROBIC ACTIVITY

30 minutes of fast walking, stationary bike, or any other type of aerobic activity that you like at your target heart rate.

14-Day Body Sculpting Workout #2

SPECIAL INSTRUCTIONS FOR WEEKS 5 & 6

Use giant sets. Perform giant sets by performing four exercises with no rest period in between. Only rest after the four exercises have been performed consecutively. Repeat for the prescribed number of sets and then move on to the second group of exercises.

DAY 1

Giant set # 1

Back—Dumbbell Rows   138
(one arm, alternate with two arms
on the next workout)
Reps: 8-10   Sets: 4
Rest: No rest

Chest—Incline Dumbbell Press   160
(alternate with Push-ups, 172)
Reps: 8-10   Sets: 4
Rest: No rest

Back—Dumbbell Pullovers   150
Reps: 8-10   Sets: 4
Rest: No rest

Chest—Incline Dumbbell Flys   166
(alternate with Push-ups, 172)
Reps: 8-10   Sets: 4
Rest: 60 seconds

Giant set # 2

Biceps—Dumbbell Curls   212
Reps: 8-10   Sets: 4
Rest: No rest

Triceps—Lying Dumbbell Extensions 194
Reps: 8-10   Sets: 4
Rest: No rest

Biceps—Concentration Curls   218
(alternate with Hammer Curls, 222)
Reps: 8-10   Sets: 4
Rest: No rest

Triceps—Triceps Kickbacks   208
(alternate with Overhead Dumbbell
Extensions, 192)
Reps: 8-10   Sets: 4
Rest: 60 seconds

DAY 2

Giant set # 1

Thighs—Dumbbell Squats   104
(alternate with Ballet Squats, 106)
Reps: 8-10   Sets: 4
Rest: No rest

Hamstrings—Lying Leg Curls   114
(alternate with Dumbbell Lunges, 108)
Reps: 8-10   Sets: 4
Rest: No rest

Thighs—Ballet Squats   106
(alternate with Leg Extensions, 112)
Reps: 8-10   Sets: 4
Rest: No rest

Hamstrings—Stiff-legged Deadlifts 120
(alternate with Standing Leg Curls, 118)
Reps: 8-10   Sets: 4
Rest: 60 seconds

Giant set # 2

Calves—Standing Calf Raises   124
(one leg)
Reps: 15-25   Sets: 4
Rest: No rest

Shoulders—Dumbbell Shoulder
Press   178
(alternate with Upright Rows, 184)
Reps: 15-25   Sets: 4
Rest: No rest

Calves—Standing Calf Raises   124
(two legs)
Reps: 15-25   Sets: 4
Rest: No rest

Shoulders—Bent-Over Lateral
Raises   186
Reps: 15-25   Sets: 4
Rest: 60 seconds

Weeks 5 & 6

DAY 3

Giant set # 1

Lower Abs—*Leg Raises*   232
Reps: 15-25   Sets: 4
Rest: No Rest

Upper Abs—*Crunches*   228
Reps: 15-25   Sets: 4
Rest: No Rest

(**Note:** Continue until all four sets of each exercise have
been done. Don't worry if you are not able to perform all of
the recommended reps the first few times you perform this
abdominal workout. As you get used to this rigorous workout, your body will adapt and get stronger).

AEROBIC ACTIVITY

40 minutes of fast walking, stationary bike, or any
other type of aerobic activity that you like at your
target heart rate.

14-Day Advanced Workout

SPECIAL INSTRUCTIONS FOR WEEKS 1 & 2

Use modified compound supersets. Perform Modified Compound Supersets by performing the first exercise, resting for the prescribed rest period, performing the second exercise, resting the prescribed rest period and going back to the first exercise. Continue in this manner until you have performed all of the prescribed number of sets. Then continue with the next modified compound superset.

DAY 1

Modified Compound Superset # 1
Back—Dumbbell Rows   138
*(one arm, alternate with two arms
on the next workout)*
Reps: 12-15   Sets: 3
Rest: 90 seconds
Chest—Incline Dumbbell Press   160
*(alternate with Incline Dumbbell Press;
palms facing each other)*
Reps: 12-15   Sets: 3
Rest: 90 seconds

Modified Compound Superset # 2
Back—Dumbbell Pullovers   150
*(alternate with Seated Low-Pulley
Rows, 148)*
Reps: 12-15   Sets: 3
Rest: 90 seconds
Chest—Chest Dips   168
(alternate with Push-ups, 172)
Reps: 12-15   Sets: 3
Rest: 90 seconds

Modified Compound Superset # 3
Back—Wide-grip Pull-ups
(or Pull-downs) to Front   140
(alternate with Wide-grip Pull-downs, 144)
Reps: 12-15   Sets: 3
Rest: 90 seconds
Chest—Incline Dumbbell Flys   166
*(alternate with Incline Cable
Crossovers, 170)*
Reps: 12-15   Sets: 3
Rest: 90 seconds

Modified Compound Superset # 4
Shoulders—Bent-Over Lateral Raises 186
(alternate with Seated Rear-Delt Machine, 188)
Reps: 12-15   Sets: 3
Rest: 90 seconds

Calves—Seated Calf Raises   122
(alternate with Donkey Calf Raises, 128)
Reps: 15-25   Sets: 3
Rest: 90 seconds

DAY 2

Modified Compound Superset # 1
Biceps—Dumbbell Curls   212
(alternate with Incline Dumbbell Curls, 214)
Reps: 12-15   Sets: 3
Rest: 90 seconds
Triceps—Lying Dumbbell Extensions 194
(alternate with Triceps Pushdowns, 206)
Reps: 12-15   Sets: 3
Rest: 90 seconds

Modified Compound Superset # 2
Biceps—Concentration Curls   218
(alternate with Hammer Curls, 222)
Reps: 12-15   Sets: 3
Rest: 90 seconds
Triceps—Triceps Kickbacks   208
*(alternate with Overhead Dumbbell
Extensions, 192)*
Reps: 12-15   Sets: 3
Rest: 90 seconds

Modified Compound Superset # 3
Biceps—Reverse Curls   224
*(alternate with One-Arm Preacher
Curls, 217)*
Reps: 12-15   Sets: 3
Rest: 90 seconds
Triceps—Triceps Dips   198
(alternate with Close-Grip Dumbbell Press, 204)
Reps: 12-15   Sets: 3
Rest: 90 seconds

Weeks 1 & 2

Modified Compound Superset # 4
Shoulders—*Dumbbell Shoulder Press* 178
(alternate with Military Press, 182)
Reps: 12-15   Sets: 3
Rest: 90 seconds
Shoulders—*Upright Rows*   184
*(alternate with Dumbbell Lateral
Raises, 180)*
Reps: 12-15   Sets: 3
Rest: 90 seconds

DAY 3

Modified Compound Superset # 1
Thighs—*Barbell Squats*   102
(alternate with Ballet Squats, 106)
Reps: 12-15   Sets: 3
Rest: 90 seconds
Hamstrings—*Lying Leg Curls*   114
(alternate with Dumbbell Lunges, 108)
Reps: 12-15   Sets: 3
Rest: 90 seconds

Modified Compound Superset # 2
Thighs—*Dumbbell Lunges*   108
(alternate with Leg Extensions, 112)
Reps: 12-15   Sets: 3
Rest: 90 seconds
Hamstrings—*Stiff-legged Deadlifts* 120
(alternate with Seated Leg Curls, 116)
Reps: 12-15   Sets: 3
Rest: 90 seconds

Modified Compound Superset # 3
Thighs—*Leg Press*   110
(alternate with Dumbbell Squats, 104)
Reps: 12-15   Sets: 3
Rest: 90 seconds
Hamstrings—*Standing Leg Curls*   118
(alternate with Lying Leg Curls, 114)
Reps: 12-15   Sets: 3
Rest: 90 seconds

Modified Compound Superset # 4
Calves—*Calf Press*   130
*(alternate with Standing Two-Legged
Calf Raises, 124)*
Reps: 15-25   Sets: 3
Rest: 90 seconds
Calves—*Standing One-Legged Calf
Raises*   124
*(alternate with Standing Two Legged
Calf Raises, 124)*
Reps: 15-25   Sets: 3
Rest: 90 seconds

CARDIO AND ABS

To be performed from Monday through Saturday first thing
in the morning on an empty stomach.

Modified Compound Superset # 1
Lower Abs—*Leg Raises*   232
Reps: 15-25   Sets: 3
Rest: 90 seconds
Upper Abs—*Crunches*   228
Reps: 15-25   Sets: 3
Rest: 90 seconds

Modified Compound Superset # 2
Lower Abs—*Knee-Ins*   236
Reps: 15-25   Sets: 3
Rest: 90 seconds
Upper Abs—*V-Ups*   230
Reps: 15-25   Sets: 3
Rest: 90 seconds

AEROBIC ACTIVITY

20 minutes of fast walking, stationary bike, or any
other type of aerobic activity that you like at your
target heart rate.

14-Day Advanced Workout

SPECIAL INSTRUCTIONS FOR WEEKS 3 & 4

Use supersets. Perform supersets by pairing exercises with no rest period in between. Only rest after the two exercises have been performed consecutively. Repeat for the prescribed number of sets and then move on to the next pair of exercises.

DAY 1

Superset # 1
Back—Dumbbell Rows   138
(one arm, alternate with two arms)
Reps: 10-12   Sets: 4
Rest: No Rest
Chest—Incline Dumbbell Press   160
(alternate with Incline Dumbbell Press;
palms facing you)
Reps: 10-12   Sets: 4
Rest: 60 seconds

Superset # 2
Back—Dumbbell Pullovers   150
(alternate with Seated Low-Pulley
Rows, 148)
Reps: 10-12   Sets: 4
Rest: No Rest
Chest—Chest Dips   168
(alternate with Push-ups, 172)
Reps: 10-12   Sets: 4
Rest: 60 seconds

Superset # 3
Back—Wide-grip Pull-ups
(or Pull-downs) to Front   140
(alternate with Wide-grip Pull-downs, 144)
Reps: 10-12   Sets: 4
Rest: No Rest
Chest—Incline Dumbbell Flys   166
(alternate with Incline Cable
Crossovers, 170)
Reps: 10-12   Sets: 4
Rest: 60 seconds

Superset # 4
Shoulders—Bent-Over Lateral Raises 186
(alternate with Seated Rear-Delt
Machine, 188)
Reps: 10-12   Sets: 4
Rest: No Rest

Calves—Seated Calf Raises   112
(alternate with Donkey Calf Raises, 128)
Reps: 15-25   Sets: 4
Rest: 60 seconds

DAY 2

Superset # 1
Biceps—Dumbbell Curls   212
(alternate with Incline Dumbbell Curls, 214)
Reps: 10-12   Sets: 4
Rest: No Rest
Triceps—Lying Dumbbell Extensions 194
(alternate with Triceps Pushdowns, 206)
Reps: 10-12   Sets: 4
Rest: 60 seconds

Superset # 2
Biceps—Concentration Curls   218
(alternate with Hammer Curls, 222)
Reps: 10-12   Sets: 4
Rest: No Rest
Triceps—Triceps Kickbacks   208
(alternate with Overhead Dumbbell
Extensions, 192)
Reps: 10-12   Sets: 4
Rest: 60 seconds

Superset # 3
Biceps—Reverse Curls   224
(alternate with One-Arm Preacher
Curls, 217)
Reps: 10-12   Sets: 4
Rest: No Rest
Triceps—Triceps Dips   198
(alternate with Close-Grip Dumbbell
Press, 204)
Reps: 10-12   Sets: 4
Rest: 60 seconds

Weeks 3 & 4

Superset # 4
Shoulders—Dumbbell Shoulder Press 178
(alternate with Military Press, 182)
Reps: 10-12   Sets: 4
Rest: No Rest
Shoulders—Upright Rows   184
(alternate with Dumbbell Lateral
Raises, 180)
Reps: 10-12   Sets: 4
Rest: 60 seconds

DAY 3

Superset # 1
Thighs—Barbell Squats   102
(alternate with Ballet Squats, 106)
Reps: 10-12   Sets: 4
Rest: No Rest
Hamstrings—Lying Leg Curls   114
(alternate with Dumbbell Lunges, 108)
Reps: 10-12   Sets: 4
Rest: 60 seconds

Superset # 2
Thighs—Dumbbell Lunges   108
(alternate with Leg Extensions, 112)
Reps: 10-12   Sets: 4
Rest: No Rest
Hamstrings—Stiff-legged Deadlifts 120
(alternate with Seated Leg Curls, 116)
Reps: 10-12   Sets: 4
Rest: 60 seconds

Superset # 3
Thighs—Leg Press   110
(alternate with Dumbbell Squats, 104)
Reps: 10-12   Sets: 4
Rest: No Rest
Hamstrings—Standing Leg Curls   118
(alternate with Lying Leg Curls, 114)
Reps: 10-12   Sets: 4
Rest: 60 seconds

Superset # 4
Calves—Calf Press   130
(alternate with Standing Two-Legged
Calf Raises, 124)
Reps: 15-25   Sets: 4
Rest: No Rest
Calves—Standing One-Legged Calf
Raises   124
(alternate with Standing Two-Legged
Calf Raises, 124)
Reps: 15-25   Sets: 4
Rest: 60 seconds

CARDIO AND ABS

To be performed from Monday through Saturday first thing in the morning on an empty stomach.

Superset # 1
Lower Abs—Leg Raises   232
Reps: 15-25   Sets: 4
Rest: No Rest
Upper Abs—Crunches   228
Reps: 15-25   Sets: 4
Rest: 60 seconds

Superset # 2
Lower Abs—Knee-Ins   236
Reps: 15-25   Sets: 4
Rest: No Rest
Upper Abs—V-Ups   230
Reps: 15-25   Sets: 4
Rest: 60 seconds

AEROBIC ACTIVITY

30 minutes of fast walking, stationary bike, or any other type of aerobic activity that you like at the target heart rate.

14-Day Advanced Workout

SPECIAL INSTRUCTIONS FOR WEEKS 5 & 6

Use giant sets. Perform giant sets by performing four exercises with no rest period in between. Only rest after the four exercises have been performed consecutively. **Repeat for** the prescribed number of sets and then move on to the second group of exercises.

DAY 1

Giant set # 1

Back—Dumbbell Rows 138
(one arm, alternate with two arms on the next workout)
Reps: 8-10   Sets: 5
Rest: No Rest

Chest—Incline Dumbbell Press 160
(alternate with Incline Dumbbell Press; palms facing you)
Reps: 8-10   Sets: 5
Rest: No Rest

Back—Dumbbell Pullovers 150
(alternate with Seated Low-Pulley Rows, 148)
Reps: 8-10   Sets: 5
Rest: No Rest

Chest—Chest Dips 168
(alternate with Push-ups, 172)
Reps: 8-10   Sets: 5
Rest: 60 seconds

Giant set # 2

Back—Wide-grip Pull-ups
(or Pull-downs) to Front 140
(alternate with Wide-grip Pull-downs, 144)
Reps: 8-10   Sets: 5
Rest: No Rest

Chest—Incline Dumbbell Flys 166
(alternate with Incline Cable Crossovers, 170)
Reps: 8-10   Sets: 5
Rest: No Rest

Shoulders—Bent-Over Lateral Raises 186
(alternate with Seated Rear-Delt Machine, 188)
Reps: 8-10   Sets: 5
Rest: No Rest

Calves—Seated Calf Raises 112
(alternate with Donkey Calf Raises, 128)
Reps: 15-25   Sets: 5
Rest: 60 seconds

DAY 2

Giant set # 1

Biceps—Dumbbell Curls 212
(alternate with Incline Dumbbell Curls, 214)
Reps: 8-10   Sets: 5
Rest: No Rest

Triceps—Lying Dumbbell Extensions 194
(alternate with Triceps Pushdowns, 206)
Reps: 8-10   Sets: 5
Rest: No Rest

Biceps—Concentration Curls 218
(alternate with Hammer Curls, 222)
Reps: 8-10   Sets: 5
Rest: No Rest

Triceps—Triceps Kickbacks 208
(alternate with Overhead Dumbbell Extensions, 192)
Reps: 8-10   Sets: 5
Rest: 60 seconds

Giant set # 2

Biceps—Reverse Curls 224
(alternate with One-Arm Preacher Curls, 217)
Reps: 8-10   Sets: 5
Rest: No Rest

Triceps—Triceps Dips 198
(alternate with Close-Grip Dumbbell Press, 204)
Reps: 8-10   Sets: 5
Rest: No Rest

Shoulders—Upright Rows 184
(alternate with Dumbbell Lateral Raises, 180)
Reps: 8-10   Sets: 5
Rest: No Rest

Shoulders—Dumbbell Shoulder Press 178
(alternate with Military Press, 182)
Reps: 8-10   Sets: 5
Rest: 60 seconds

Weeks 5 & 6

DAY 3

Giant set # 1

Thighs—*Barbell Squats*   102
(alternate with Ballet Squats, 106)
Reps: 8-10   Sets: 5
Rest: No Rest

Hamstrings—*Lying Leg Curls*   114
(alternate with Dumbbell Lunges, 108)
Reps: 8-10   Sets: 5
Rest: No Rest

Thighs—*Dumbbell Lunges*   108
(alternate with Leg Extensions, 112)
Reps: 8-10   Sets: 5
Rest: No Rest

Hamstrings—*Standing Leg Curls*   118
(alternate with Lying Leg Curls, 114)
Reps: 8-10   Sets: 5
Rest: 60 seconds

Giant set # 2

Thighs—*Leg Press*   110
(alternate with Dumbbell Squats, 104)
Reps: 8-10   Sets: 5
Rest: No Rest

Hamstrings—*Stiff-legged Deadlifts*   120
(alternate with Seated Leg Curls, 116)
Reps: 8-10   Sets: 5
Rest: No Rest

Calves—*Calf Press*   130
*(alternate with Standing Two-Legged
Calf Raises, 124)*
Reps: 15-25   Sets: 5
Rest: No Rest

Calves—*Standing One-Legged Calf
Raises*   124
*(alternate with Standing Two-Legged
Calf Raises, 124)*
Reps: 15-25   Sets: 5
Rest: 60 seconds

CARDIO AND ABS

To be performed from Monday through Saturday first thing in the morning on an empty stomach.

Giant set # 1

Lower Abs—*Leg Raises*   232
Reps: 15-25   Sets: 5
Rest: No Rest

Upper Abs—*Crunches*   228
Reps: 15-25   Sets: 5
Rest: 60 seconds

Lower Abs—*Knee-Ins*   236
Reps: 15-25   Sets: 5
Rest: No Rest

Upper Abs—*V-Ups*   230
Reps: 15-25   Sets: 5
Rest: 60 seconds

AEROBIC ACTIVITY

40 minutes of fast walking, stationary bike, or any other type of aerobic activity that you like at your target heart rate.

14-Day Body Sculpting Mass

SPECIAL INSTRUCTIONS FOR WEEKS 1 & 2

Use Modified Compound Supersets. Perform these sets by competing the first set of the first exercise, resting for the pre-scribed rest period, performing the first set of the second exercise, resting the prescribed rest period, and then doing the second set of the first exercise. Continue in this manner until you have completed all of the prescribed number of sets for each exercise. Then move on to the next Modified Compound Superset.

DAY 1

Modified Compound Superset # 1
Back—*Dumbbell Rows (one arm)*　　138
Reps: 10-12　　　Sets: 3
Rest: 90 seconds
Chest—*Incline Dumbbell Press*　　160
Reps: 10-12　　　Sets: 3
Rest: 90 seconds

Modified Compound Superset # 2
Back—*Wide Grip Pull-ups to Front*　140
Reps: 10-12　　　Sets: 2
Rest: 90 seconds
Chest—*Chest Dips*　　168
Reps: 10-12　　　Sets: 2
Rest: 90 seconds

Modified Compound Superset # 3
Biceps—*Standing E-Z Bar Curls*　　220
Reps: 10-12　　　Sets: 3
Rest: 90 seconds
Triceps—*Lying E-Z Bar Extensions*　196
Reps: 10-12　　　Sets: 3
Rest: 90 seconds

Modified Compound Superset # 4
Biceps—*Hammer Curls*　　222
Reps: 10-12　　　Sets: 2
Rest: 90 seconds
Triceps—*Overhead Dumbbell
Extensions*　　192
Reps: 10-12　　　Sets: 2
Rest: 90 seconds

DAY 2

Modified Compound Superset # 1
Thighs—*Leg Press*　　110
Reps: 10-12　　　Sets: 3
Rest: 90 seconds
Hamstrings—*Seated Leg Curls*　　116
Reps: 10-12　　　Sets: 3
Rest: 90 seconds

Modified Compound Superset # 2
Thighs—*Dumbbell Lunges*　　108
Reps: 10-12　　　Sets: 2
Rest: 90 seconds
Hamstrings—*Stiff-Legged Deadlifts*　120
Reps: 10-12　　　Sets: 2
Rest: 90 seconds

Modified Compound Superset # 3
Calves—*Standing Calf Raises
(one leg)*　　124
Reps: 12-15　　　Sets: 3
Rest: 90 seconds
Shoulders—*Dumbbell Shoulder
Press*　　178
Reps: 10-12　　　Sets: 3
Rest: 90 seconds

Modified Compound Superset # 4
Calves—*Standing Calf Raises
(two legs)*　　124
Reps: 12-15　　　Sets: 2
Rest: 90 seconds
Shoulders—*Bent-Over Lateral Raises*　186
Reps: 10-12　　　Sets: 2
Rest: 90 seconds

Workout

Weeks 1 & 2

DAY 3

Modified Compound Superset # 1

Lower Abs—*Leg Raises*   232
Reps: 10-12   Sets: 3
Rest: 90 seconds

Upper Abs— *Crunches*   228
Reps: 10-12   Sets: 2
Rest: 90 seconds

AEROBIC ACTIVITY

20 minutes of fast walking, stationary bike, or any other type of aerobic activity that you prefer at the target heart rate.

14-Day Body Sculpting Mass

SPECIAL INSTRUCTIONS FOR WEEKS 3 & 4

Use supersets. Perform these sets by pairing exercises with no rest period in between. Rest only after the two exercises have been performed consecutively. Repeat this routine for the prescribed number of sets before moving on to the next pair of exercises.

DAY 1

Superset # 1
Back—Close Grip Pull-up   142
Reps: 8-10   Sets: 4
Rest: No Rest
Chest—Flat Dumbbell Press   162
Reps: 8-10   Sets: 4
Rest: 60 seconds

Superset # 2
Back—Bent-Over Barbell Row   136
Reps: 8-10   Sets: 3
Rest: No Rest
Chest— Flat Dumbbell Press   162
Reps: 8-10   Sets: 3
Rest: 60 seconds

Superset # 3
Biceps—Incline Dumbbell Curl   214
Reps: 8-10   Sets: 4
Rest: No Rest
Triceps—Close-Grip Dumbbell Press 204
Reps: 8-10   Sets: 4
Rest: 60 seconds

Superset # 4
Biceps—Reverse Curl   224
Reps: 8-10   Sets: 3
Rest: No Rest
Triceps—Triceps Pushdown   206
Reps: 8-10   Sets: 3
Rest: 60 seconds

DAY 2

Superset # 1
Thighs—Close Stance Barbell Squat 102
Reps: 8-10   Sets: 4
Rest: No Rest
Hamstrings—Lying Leg Curl   114
Reps: 8-10   Sets: 4
Rest: 60 seconds

Superset # 2
Thighs—Leg Extension   112
Reps: 8-10
Sets: 3   Rest: No Rest
Hamstrings—Leg Press   110
Reps: 8-10   Sets: 3
Rest: 60 seconds

Superset # 3
Calves-Standing Machine Calf Raise 124
Reps: 12-15   Sets: 4
Rest: No Rest
Shoulders—Upright Row   184
Reps: 8-10   Sets: 4
Rest: 60 seconds

Superset # 4
Calves—Seated Machine Calf Raise 126
Reps: 12-15   Sets: 3
Rest: No Rest
Shoulders—Bent Over Lateral Raise 186
Reps: 8-10   Sets: 3
Rest: 60 seconds

Workout

DAY 3

Superset # 1
Lower Abs*—Leg Raises*   232
Reps: 10-12   Sets: 4
Rest: No Rest
Upper Abs*—Crunches*   228
Reps: 10-12   Sets: 3
Rest: 60 seconds

AEROBIC ACTIVITY

25 minutes of fast walking, stationary bike, or any other type of aerobic activity that you prefer at your target heart rate.

14-Day Body Sculpting Mass

SPECIAL INSTRUCTIONS FOR WEEKS 5 & 6

Use Giant Sets. Perform these sets by doing four exercises with no rest periods in between. Rest only after the four exercises have been performed consecutively. Repeat for the prescribed number of sets before moving on to the next group of exercises.

DAY 1

Giantset # 1

Back—*Narrow-Grip Pull-down*   146
Reps: 6-8   Sets: 4
Rest: No rest

Chest—*Incline Dumbbell Press*   160
Reps: 6-8   Sets: 4
Rest: No rest

Back—*Dumbbell Rows*   138
Reps: 6-8   Sets: 4
Rest: No rest

Chest—*Flat Dumbbell Press*   162
Reps: 6-8   Sets: 4
Rest: 60 seconds

Giantset # 2

Biceps—*One-Arm Preacher Curls*   216
Reps: 8-10   Sets: 4
Rest: No rest

Triceps—*Triceps Dips*   198
Reps: 8-10   Sets: 4
Rest: No rest

Biceps—*Reverse Curl*   224
Reps: 8-10   Sets: 4
Rest: No rest

Triceps—*E-Z Curl Bar Close-Grip
Press*   202
Reps: 8-10   Sets: 4
Rest: 60 seconds

DAY 2

Giantset # 1

Thighs—*Barbell Squats*   102
Reps: 6-8   Sets: 4
Rest: No rest

Hamstrings—*Barbell Lunges*   108
Reps: 6-8   Sets: 4
Rest: No rest

Thighs—*Ballet Squats*   107
Reps: 6-8   Sets: 4
Rest: No rest

Hamstrings—*Barbell Stiff-legged
Deadlifts*   120
Reps: 6-8   Sets: 4
Rest: 60 seconds

Giantset # 2

Calves—*Calf Press*   130
Reps: 6-8   Sets: 4
Rest: No rest

Shoulders—*Military Press*   182
Reps: 6-8   Sets: 4
Rest: No rest

Calves—*Donkey Calf Raises*   128
Reps: 6-8   Sets: 4
Rest: No rest

Shoulders—*Seated Rear Delt-
Machine*   188
Reps: 6-8   Sets: 4
Rest: 60 seconds

Workout

Weeks 5 & 6

DAY 3

Giantset # 1

Lower Abs—*Leg Raises*   *232*
Reps: 10-12   Sets: 4
Rest: No Rest

Upper Abs—*Crunches*   *228*
Reps: 10-12   Sets: 4
Rest: No Rest

(Note: Continue until you complete all four sets of each exercise. Don't worry if the first few times that you perform this abdominal workout you are not able to perform all of the recommended reps . As you get used to this rigorous workout, your body will adapt and become stronger.)

AEROBIC ACTIVITY

30 minutes of fast walking, stationary bike, or any other type of aerobic activity that you prefer at your target heart rate.

Appendix A
Glossary

A

Aerobic Exercise: Constant moderate intensity work that uses oxygen at a rate in which the cardio respiratory system can replenish oxygen in the working muscles. Examples of such activity are stationary bike riding or walking. It is a good activity for fat loss when done in the right amounts but highly catabolic if done in excess.

Anaerobic Exercise: Exercise in which oxygen is used more quickly than the body is able to replenish it inside the working muscle. Weight training is an example of such an activity. It is highly anabolic in nature but also highly catabolic if done in excess.

Anabolic State: Favorable state in the body created by a combination of good training, nutrition and rest that leads to favorable changes in body composition.

Anabolic Steroids: Synthetic (man-made) hormones that simulate the effects of the male hormone testosterone.

Anti-catabolic Properties: Properties provided by certain nutrients that protect the muscle mass in the body from being broken down.

Anti-lypolitic Properties: Properties provided by certain nutrients that prevent the body from turning calories into fat.

Antioxidant Properties: Properties provided by certain nutrients that protect the body from disease.

Basic Exercises: Exercise movement that involves a large number of muscles in the body. They are generally multi-joint movements that target the larger muscles of the body (such as chest, back and thighs) but also involve the smaller muscles as well (such as

shoulders, arms, calves and abs) as auxiliary muscles. Examples of such movements are chin-ups, pull-ups, dips, bench presses, squats, and lunges.

Bulk Minerals: Minerals which the body needs in great quantities (in the order of grams) such as calcium, magnesium, potassium, sodium and phosphorus.

Carbohydrates: Macronutrient used by the body as its main source of energy. Carbohydrates are divided into complex carbs and simple carbs. The complex carbs give you sustained energy ("timed release") while the simple carbs give you immediate energy. This macronutrient can be found in rice (complex, starchy), pasta (complex, starchy), breads (complex, starchy), fruits (simple), sugars (simple), fruit juices (simple), dairy products (simple), and vegetables (complex, fibrous).

Catabolic State: Unfavorable state in the body created by a combination of too much training, lack of good nutrition and lack of rest that leads to muscle loss and fat accumulation.

Cortisol: Catabolic hormone secreted by the adrenal glands in situations of stress (both physical and mental), lack of calories/nutrients and lack of sleep. This hormone is associated with loss of muscle mass, loss of strength, and fat accumulation. An excess of it over long periods of time may also contribute to hardening of the arteries; leading to heart disease.

Diuretics: Drugs used to remove excess water from the body. There are two versions: the drug version (can only be prescribed by a physician), and the herbal version. Excessive use of the drug version has as side effects muscle cramps and harsh arrhythmia. The herbal version, while safer than the drug version, can lead to potassium loss and excessive use puts stress on the kidneys.

Dumbbell: A short-handled barbell 10-12 inches long that can be carried in one hand. Dumbbells allow flexibility in the execution of a movement and full range of motion.

Endorphins: Hormones that make us feel good and happy. The production of these hormones is stimulated by exercise.

Essential Fatty Acids (EFAs): Fats that have anti-catabolic, anti-lypolitic and antioxidant properties. These fats affect good cholesterol in a positive way. In addition, these fats aid in the muscle-building, fat-loss process. The Omega 3 Fatty Acids found in fats such as fish oils and flaxseed oil are a good source of EFAs.

Estrogen: Female hormone that regulates and sustains female sexual development and reproductive function. An excess of this hormone appears to be related to heart disease and cancer. In addition, when this hormone is in excess, it causes fat gain and water retention. Estrogen deficits, on the other hand, cause memory problems, trouble finding words, inability to pay attention, mood swings and irritability. Exercise reduces the risk of these diseases and conditions by helping to balance the levels of this hormone.

Exercise Volume: The amount of work performed in an exercise session defined by the product resulting from the amount of weight lifted, multiplied by the number of sets and multiplied by the number of repetitions. For example, if you had a workout that consisted of 10 sets of dumbbell curls, and for each set you used 30 pounds and performed 10 repetitions, then your biceps routine volume equals

10 x 10 x 30=3000 pounds. Too much volume leads to overtraining.

Fats: Macronutrient needed by the body in order to manufacture hormones and sustain cell metabolism. All the cells in the body have some fat in them. Hormones are manufactured from fats. Also, fats lubricate your joints. If you eliminate the fat from your diet, your hormonal production will go down and a whole array of chemical reactions will be interrupted. There are three types of fats: saturated, polyunsaturated and monounsaturated.

Fat Soluble Vitamins: Vitamins stored in fat that if taken in excessive amounts will become toxic. They include vitamins A, D, E, and K.

Giant Set: Giant Sets are four exercises done one after the other with no rest in between sets. Again, there are two ways to implement this. You can either use four exercises for the same muscle group or perform two pairs of opposing muscle group exercises. For the purposes of this manual, whenever we do Giant Sets, we will perform two pairs of opposing muscle group exercises with no rest. The exception is when we do Abs in which we will alternate between lower abs and upper abs.

Growth Hormone: Hormone secreted by the pituitary gland that aids in fat loss and muscle building.

Hormones: Fats similar to, and usually synthesized from, cholesterol, starting with Acetyl-CoA, moving through squalene, lanosterol, cholesterol, and, in the gonads and adrenal cortex, a number of steroid hormones. Because they stimulate cell growth, either by changing the internal structure or increasing the rate of proliferation, they are often called anabolic steroids.

Hypertrophy: Scientific term for describing an increase in muscle mass and strength caused by the stimulation of the muscles.

Intensity: Intensity has two definitions in the weight-training world. (1) Relative term that indicates the level of effort exerted during the performance of an exercise. (2) In strength training circles, intensity refers to the amount of weight used on a specific exercise.

Insulin: Hormone secreted by the pancreas responsible for carbohydrate metabolism. This hormone determines if carbohydrates are to be used for energy, storage inside the muscle cells as glycogen, or converting and storing the carbohydrates as fats when they are found in excess in the bloodstream.

Isolation Exercises: Exercise movements that are generally single jointed and serve to isolate a single area of the body. Examples of such are dumbbell flys, concentration curls, triceps kickbacks, leg extensions, and leg curls.

Lactic Acid: By-product created by a lack of oxygen flow to the working muscles. Lactic acid is created by anaerobic activities such as weight training exercises. It is believed that its presence causes a surge in growth hormone levels.

Macronutrient: One of the three major nutrients that the body needs for survival. These nutrients are carbohydrates, proteins and fats.

Metabolism: The rate at which the body utilizes calories and nutrients in order to sustain its daily activities.

Minerals: Minerals are inorganic compounds (not produced by animals or vegetables) whose main function is to assure that your brain receives the correct signals from the body, as well as to ensure balance of fluids, make muscular contractions possible and allow energy production, as well as building muscle and bones. There are two types of minerals: bulk and trace minerals.

Modified Compound Superset: In a modified compound set, you pair exercises for opposing muscle groups or for opposing muscle movements (e.g. Push vs. Pull). First you perform one exercise, rest the recommended amount of seconds and then perform the second exercise (for instance, first do biceps, rest, then do triceps). You then rest the prescribed amount of time again and go back to the first exercise. Using this technique of pairing exercises in a modified superset fashion not only saves time and keeps the body warm, but allows for faster recovery of the nervous system between sets. This will allow the person to lift heavier weights than possible if he just stayed idle for 2-3 minutes waiting to recover.

Monounsaturated Fats: Fats that have a positive effect on good cholesterol levels. These fats are usually high in essential fatty acids and may have antioxidant properties. Sources of these fats are fish oils, virgin olive oil, canola oil, and flaxseed oil.

Muscle Failure: Point during the exercise at which it becomes impossible to perform another repetition in good form. This point is reached due to the lack of oxygen reaching the working muscles and the increased levels of lactic acid.

Overtraining: Condition caused by an excess of volume in a training routine that leads to muscle loss, strength loss and fat accumulation. Symptoms include depression, insomnia, lethargy and lack of energy.

Polyunsaturated Fats: Fats that do not have an affect on cholesterol levels. Most of the fats in vegetable oils, such as corn, cottonseed, safflower, soybean, and sunflower oil are polyunsaturated.

Protein: Every tissue in your body is made from protein (i.e. muscle, hair, skin, nails). Proteins are the building blocks of muscle tissue. This macronutrient can be found in poultry, meats, and dairy products.

Repetitions: The amount of times you perform an exercise. For instance, pretend that you are performing a bench press. You pick up the bar, lower it, pause and lift it up. That action of executing the movement for one time counts for one repetition. If you perform that same movement a second time, then that is your second repetition, and so on.

Rest Interval: The amount of time a person rests between sets. For instance, a rest interval of 60 seconds means that after you finish your first set, you will remain idle for 60 seconds before going on to the next set.

Saturated Fats: Saturated fats are associated with heart disease and high cholesterol levels. They are found to a large extent in products of animal origin. However, some vegetable fats are altered in a way that increases the amount of saturated fats in them by a chemical process known as hydrogenation. Hydrogenated vegetable oils are generally found in packaged foods. In addition, coconut oil, palm oil, and palm kernel oil, which are also frequently used in packaged foods and non-dairy creamers are also highly saturated.

Sets: A set is a collection of repetitions that culminates in the muscle reaching muscular failure.

Supersets: A superset is a combination of one exercise performed right after the other with no rest in between. There are two ways to implement a superset. The first way is to do two exercises for the same muscle group at once; for example dumbbell curls immediately followed by concentration curls. The drawback to this technique is that you will not be as strong as you usually are on the second exercise. The second and best way to superset is by pairing exercises of opposing muscle groups or different muscle movements such as back and chest, thighs and hamstrings, biceps and triceps, shoulders and calves, upper abs and lower abs. When pairing antagonistic exercises, there is no drop of strength once your cardiovascular system is well conditioned.

Trace Minerals: Minerals which are needed by the body in minute amounts, usually in the order of micrograms, such as chromium, copper, cobalt, silicon, selenium, iron and zinc.

Testosterone: Hormone responsible for increasing muscle size. Even though this hormone is predominantly present in males, it is also present in women to a lesser degree. It is believed that this hormone also aids in fat loss to a lesser degree.

Vitamins: Vitamins are organic compounds (produced by both animals and vegetables) whose function is to enhance the actions of proteins that cause chemical reactions such as muscle building, fat burning and energy production. There are two types of vitamins: fat-soluble and water-soluble.

Water Soluble Vitamins: Vitamins that are not stored in the body, such as B-Complex vitamins and vitamin C. Therefore, they need to be taken on a frequent basis.

B

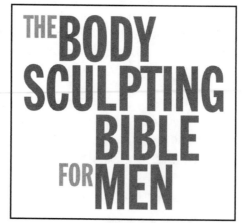

THE BODY
SCULPTING
BIBLE
FOR MEN

FOOD GROUP TABLES

For the post-workout meal (meal that comes after the workout is performed), choose 1 item from Group A and 1 item from Group C in order to create a balanced meal. For all other meals, choose 1 item from Group A, 1 item from Group B, and 1 item from Group D in order to create a balanced meal. Remember to adjust the serving size depending upon the amount of nutrients that you require per meal (remember your calculations guys? Go back and figure them out if you haven't already).

GROUP A - PROTEIN

FOOD	GRAMS	FOOD	GRAMS
Chicken breast (3.5 oz. broiled)	33	White fish (3.5 oz broiled)	31
Tuna (packed in water, 3.5 oz)	35	Halibut (3.5 oz broiled)	31
Turkey breast (3.5 oz broiled)	28	Cod (3.5 oz broiled)	31
Whey protein powder (2 scoops)	22	Round steak (3.5 oz broiled)	33
10 egg whites	35	Top sirloin (4 oz)	35

Note: These weights are for uncooked portions

GROUP B - CARBOHYDRATE (COMPLEX, STARCHY)

FOOD	GRAMS	FOOD	GRAMS
Baked potato (3.5 oz broiled)	21	Lentils (1 cup dry, cooked)	38
Plain oatmeal (1/2 cup dry)	27	Grits (1/2 cup dry)	31
Whole wheat bread (1 slice; limit if reducing body fat)	13	Pita bread (1 piece)	33
Cream of rice (1/2 cup dry, post workout only)	38	Sweet potato (4 oz)	28
Chickpeas (1 cup cooked)	45	Brown rice (2/3 cup cooked)	30

GROUP C - CARBOHYDRATE (SIMPLE)

FOOD	GRAMS	FOOD	GRAMS
Apple (1)	15	Banana (6 oz, *post workout only*)	27
Cantaloupe (1/2)	25	Grapes (1 cup, *post workout only*)	14
Strawberries (1 cup)	9	Grapefruit (1/2)	12
Orange (1)	15	Tangerine (1)	9
Pear (1)	27	Cherries (1 cup)	22
Lemon (1)	5	Nectarine (1)	16
Peach (1)	10	Skim milk (1 cup, *preferably post workout only*)	13

GROUP D - CARBOHYDRATE (COMPLEX, FIBROUS)

FOOD (10 OZ SERVING)	GRAMS	FOOD (10 OZ SERVING)	GRAMS
Asparagus	5	Yellow squash	12
Broccoli	17	Green beans	23
Cabbage	6	Cauliflower	12
Celery	6	Cucumber	7
Mushrooms	6	Lettuce	7
Red or Green peppers	15	Tomato	5
Spinach	3	Zucchini	13

NOTES:

- While the foods above contain trace amounts of other macronutrients (for example, skinless chicken breasts contain 2.5 to 5 grams of fat), for the purposes of our calculations, we will assume that these food contain only the macronutrient under which they are listed.

- Always try to use natural foods. Avoid using canned or pre-prepared types of foods as they usually contain too much fats, sodium and carbs.

- Stay within plus or minus 10 grams of the recommended amount of carbs and proteins. For fats, stay within +/- 5 grams.

- Always choose low fat protein sources. If you eat really low fat meals, don't worry about incurring into a fat deficiency since the supplements program takes care of the need for essential fatty acids. Besides, there are trace amounts of fats even in the low fat protein sources that we choose.

- If you choose to include skim milk in your diet, remember that it not only has protein (8 to 9 grams for every 8 ounces of milk) but also simple carbs (12 to 13 grams for every 8 ounces of milk). Therefore, count milk as both. Note that since the carbs in milk are simple carbs, this food item should only be used in the post workout meal. However, if due to schedule you need to include more protein shakes throughout the day, and the carbs that you will rely on are those found in skim milk, ensure that you add a teaspoon of flaxseed oil to it as the oil will slow down the release of the simple carbs into the blood stream. Guys interested in competing should however eliminate any dairy products from the diet as these products tend to make you retain water and the lactose in them make it harder to get to the desired low body fat percentage required for contest condition. In addition, whole wheat products should also be minimized during this phase as they may contain pytho-estrogens that would make it harder to lose fat.

- Try to include Fibrous Carbs in at least two meals.

- Post Workout Meal should contain high glycemic carbs combined with fast released proteins such as whey protein isolate. Fats and fibers should be eliminated from this meal.

- If you use flaxseed oil as your Essential Fatty Acids supplement, remember to count itas fat grams. Each teaspoon contains approximately 5 grams of good fats.

- If you use fish oil capsules as your Essential Fatty Acids supplement, count each capsule as 1 gram of good fats.

- Remember that carbohydrates have 4 calories per gram. Therefore, a 6-ounce banana has 27 grams of carbs x 4 = 108 calories.

- Remember that protein has 4 calories per gram. Therefore, a 3.5-ounce chicken breast has 35 grams of protein x 4 = 140 calories.

- Remember that fat has 9 calories per gram. Therefore, a teaspoon of flaxseed oil has 5 grams of fat x 9 = 45 calories.

Appendix C
Sample Diets

C

THE **BODY SCULPTING BIBLE** FOR **MEN**

The following are sample diets. You may substitute foods as long as you substitute an amount that yields approximately the same amount of macronutrients (Carbs, Protein and Fats). Note that we included many liquid meals. The reason for that is that we created the menus under the assumption that the person using them is always on the go and has no time to eat four or five real meals. However, we encourage the use of solid food as often as possible.

Also, make sure that you adjust your feeding times depending on your schedule. The requirement is that you eat every two to three hours after your first meal (ensure that your first meal is eaten by 9:30 a.m. at the latest).

Note: Always drink enough ounces of water (your bodyweight multiplied by 0.66) each day.

SAMPLE 14-DAY LOW CALORIE CYCLE DIET

MEAL #	FOOD	SERVING SIZE	CALORIES	CARBS (grams)	PROTEIN (grams)	FAT (grams)
MEAL 1 **BREAKFAST** **(POST-WORKOUT)** **9:00 AM**	Skim Milk Whey Protein 1 banana TOTALS:	24 ounces 4 scoops 6 ounces	504	34 - 26 60	26 40 - 66	- - - -
MEAL 2 **LUNCH** **12:00 NOON**	Chicken Breast White Rice Green Beans TOTALS:	6 ounces 1 cup cooked 5 ounces	472	0 45 13 58	60 - - 60	- - - -
MEAL 3 **SNACK** **3:00 PM**	Skim Milk Whey Protein Flaxseed Oil TOTALS:	24 ounces 2 scoop 1 teaspoon	377	39 - - 39	24 20 - 44	- - 5 5
MEAL 4 **DINNER** **6:00 PM**	Tuna Fish (packed in water) Baked Potato (broiled) Broccoli Flaxseed Oil TOTALS:	4 ounces 3.5 ounces 7 ounces 1 teaspoon	361	- 21 18 - 39	40 - - - 40	- - - 5 5
MEAL 5 **LATE SNACK** **8:00 PM**	Skim Milk Whey Protein Flaxseed Oil TOTALS:	16 ounces 2 scoop 1 teaspoon	293	26 - - 26	16 20 - 36	- - 5 5
DAILY TOTALS:			2007	235	254	15

SAMPLE 14-DAY HIGH CALORIE CYCLE DIET

MEAL #	FOOD	SERVING SIZE	CALORIES	CARBS (grams)	PROTEIN (grams)	FAT (grams)
MEAL 1 BREAKFAST (POST WORKOUT) 9:00 AM	Skim Milk	24 ounces	504	34	26	-
	Whey Protein	4 scoops		-	40	-
	1 banana	6 ounces		26	-	-
	TOTALS:			20	66	-
MEAL 2 LUNCH 12:00 NOON	Chicken Breast	6 ounces	472	0	60	-
	White Rice	1 cup cooked		45	-	-
	Green Beans	5 ounces		13	-	-
	TOTALS:			58	60	-
MEAL 3 SNACK 3:00PM	Skim Milk	24 ounces	377	39	24	-
	Whey Protein	2 scoops		-	20	-
	Flaxseed Oil	1 teaspoon		-	-	5
	TOTALS:			39	44	5
MEAL 4 DINNER 5:30 PM	Tuna Fish (packed in water)	4 ounces	361	-	40	-
	Baked Potato (broiled)	3.5 ounces		21	-	-
	Broccoli	7 ounces		18	-	-
	Flaxseed Oil	1 teaspoon		-	-	5
	TOTALS:			39	40	5
MEAL 5 LATE SNACK 7:30PM	White Rice	1 cup cooked	517	45	-	-
	Green Beans	5 ounces		13	-	-
	Chicken Breast	6 ounces		0	60	-
	Flaxseed Oil	1 teaspoon		-	-	5
	TOTALS:			58	60	5
MEAL 6 LATE SNACK 9:30 PM	Skim Milk	16 ounces	293	26	16	-
	Whey Protein	2 scoops		-	20	-
	Flaxseed Oil	1 teaspoon		-	-	5
	TOTALS:			26	36	5
DAILY TOTALS:			2574	293	314	20

NOTES:

- For both diets we assumed that your workout was before breakfast. If you are following The Advanced 14-Day Body Sculpting Workout, ensure that you consume another shake within 60 minutes after the weight-training workout in order to enhance recuperation and to cover your increased energy needs. This shake will add approximately another 250 calories to the totals above. In this case, you will be having seven meals a day.

- Recall that for our calculations we are assuming that the foods above (except for skim milk) do not contain any other macronutrients. However, since they do, the actual caloric intake is a bit higher; probably 100 calories higher than what we calculate above. This is okay as all we need is a reference point to begin.

- Because the low fat protein sources that we choose do have some fats in them, you need not be concerned about incurring into a fat deficiency in your diet. You will be getting the required 20% of the calories from fat when you combine the trace amounts of fats found in the protein we choose with the supplemental fat we suggest.

Appendix D
Workout Journal

THE **BODY**
SCULPTING
BIBLE
FOR **MEN**

D

BREAK-IN ROUTINE #1

Daily Workout Journal   Week ◯ Day ◯

Exercise Main (Alternate)	Rest	Set 1 Reps	Set 1 Weight	Set 2 Reps	Set 2 Weight	Set 3 Reps	Set 3 Weight	Set 4 Reps	Set 4 Weight	Set 5 Reps	Set 5 Weight
Group 1											
Group 2											
Group 3											
Group 4											
Abs											

Cardio

Cardio Activity: _____   Notes: _____

Average Heart Rate: _____

Duration: _____

Notes

BREAK-IN ROUTINE #2

Daily Workout Journal

Week ⬤ Day ⬤

	Exercise Main (Alternate)	Rest	Set 1 Reps	Weight	Set 2 Reps	Weight	Set 3 Reps	Weight	Set 4 Reps	Weight	Set 5 Reps	Weight	
Group 1													Group 1
Group 2													Group 2
Group 3													Group 3
Group 4													Group 4
Abs													Abs

Cardio		Notes
Cardio Activity:		Notes:
Average Heart Rate:		
Duration:		

14-DAY BODY SCULPTING WORKOUT #1

Daily Workout Journal

Week ◯   Day ◯

Exercise Main (Alternate)	Rest	Set 1 Reps	Weight	Set 2 Reps	Weight	Set 3 Reps	Weight	Set 4 Reps	Weight	Set 5 Reps	Weight
Group 1											
Group 2											
Group 3											
Group 4											
Abs											

Cardio

Cardio Activity: Notes:

Average Heart Rate:

Duration:

Notes

14-DAY BODY SCULPTING WORKOUT #2

Daily Workout Journal   Week ⬤ Day ⬤

	Exercise Main (Alternate)	Rest	Set 1 Reps / Weight	Set 2 Reps / Weight	Set 3 Reps / Weight	Set 4 Reps / Weight	Set 5 Reps / Weight	
Group 1								**Group 1**
Group 2								**Group 2**
Group 3								**Group 3**
Group 4								**Group 4**
Abs								**Abs**

Cardio	Cardio Activity: Notes:	**Notes**
	Average Heart Rate:	
	Duration:	

14-DAY ADVANCED WORKOUT

Daily Workout Journal   Week ◯   Day ◯

Exercise Main (Alternate)	Rest	Set 1 Reps	Set 1 Weight	Set 2 Reps	Set 2 Weight	Set 3 Reps	Set 3 Weight	Set 4 Reps	Set 4 Weight	Set 5 Reps	Set 5 Weight
Group 1											
Group 2											
Group 3											
Group 4											
Abs											

Cardio

Cardio Activity: Notes:

Average Heart Rate:

Duration:

14-DAY BODY SCULPTING MASS WORKOUT

Daily Workout Journal

Week ⬤ Day ⬤

	Exercise Main (Alternate)	Rest	Set 1		Set 2		Set 3		Set 4		Set 5		
			Reps	Weight	Reps	Weight	Reps	Weight	Reps	Weight	Reps	Weight	
Group 1													**Group 1**
Group 2													**Group 2**
Group 3													**Group 3**
Group 4													**Group 4**
Abs													**Abs**

Cardio	Cardio Activity:	Notes:	**Notes**
	Average Heart Rate:		
	Duration:		

E

THE **BODY**
SCULPTING
BIBLE
FOR**MEN**

Daily Nutrition Journal

Week ◯ Day ◯

	Food	Serving Size	Calories	Carbs (grams)	Protein (grams)	Fat (grams)
Meal 1						
Meal 2						
Meal 3						
Meal 4						
Meal 5						
Meal 6						
Total						

Tracking Your Progress

F

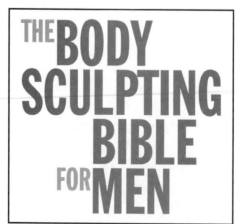

THE **BODY**
SCULPTING
BIBLE
FOR **MEN**

The only way to know if your program is working or not is by tracking your progress. A simple way to do this is by using the following formulas excerpted from the book *Hardcore Bodybuilding: A Scientific Approach,* written by strength training authority Frederick C. Hatfield, Ph.D. Dr. Hatfield, better known as Dr. Squat, is the co-founding Director of Sports and Fitness Sciences for the prestigious International Sports Sciences Association (ISSA). As a three-time winner of the World Championships of Powerlifting, Dr. Hatfield not only is well versed on weight training theory, but on its application as well.

FOR MEN:

Before you use the formulas, there are two measurements that are required:

Measurement 1: Bodyweight

Measurement 2: Waist Girth (measured at the umbilicus)

PROCEDURE:

1) Multiply your bodyweight by 1.082. Add the result to 94.42. Once your calculation is complete, save the number. ➜ (Bodyweight x 1.082) + 94.42=Result 1

2) Multiply your waist girth by 4.15. Once you get this result, subtract it from the number obtained in step 1 (ie: Step 1 result-Step 2 result). The result obtained after the subtraction is done is your lean bodyweight (your weight if you had no fat in your body at all).

➜ Result 1—(Waist Girth x 4.15)= Lean Body Weight

3) Finally, subtract your lean bodyweight from your total bodyweight (Total weight-Lean Bodyweight). Once you get the result, multiply that number by 100. Once you get the result divide it by your total bodyweight. This final result is your percentage of body fat.
➜ ((Total Bodyweight—Lean Bodyweight) x 100) divided by (Your Body Weight) = Your Percentage of Body Fat.

EXAMPLE:

I weigh 190 and I have a 30.5 inch waist. Therefore, step 1 is (190 x 1.082) + 94.42 = 300. Step 2 says that my lean body weight equals 300-(30.5 x 4.15)=173.425. Finally, Step 3 says that my body fat percentage is ((190-173.425) x 100) divided by 190= 8.72%.

Notes: The formulas above are approximations. The goal here is to have a point of reference from which to work. I recommend that you measure your body fat every three weeks. If you see a pattern where you are gaining muscle and losing fat, then you know your program is on track. If not, examine which part of your program is not optimal. Assuming that you are following the recommended training routines, then the only things that could be going wrong are either you are not getting enough rest at night, or more likely that you are not following the nutrition plan properly. You will also want to take your body fat measurements and can do so by purchasing a pair of body fat calipers. This will be a very good indicator of how much fat you are losing, much better than the mistaken theory of "weight" being the method of calculating improvements.

Grocery Shopping List

G

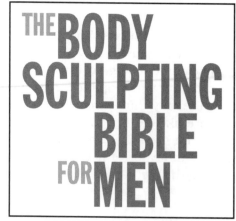

Note: Eat a meal prior to going grocery shopping to ensure that you don't buy junk foods. Another strategy is to do your grocery shopping on Sundays, when you are allowed to eat whatever you want for one meal.

Obviously, you do not need to purchase all of the items on this grocery list. We provide it as a reminder of the types of foods that your shopping list should include.

CARBOHYDRATES

- Brown rice
- Chickpeas
- Cream of rice
- Yams (sweet potatoes)
- Whole wheat bread
- Plain oatmeal (old fashion, not instant)
- Corn
- Baking potato
- Lentils
- Pita bread
- Lentils
- Grits
- Fruits
- Fresh green vegetables

PROTEINS

- Chicken breasts (avoid deli meats; they are high in sodium and low in protein)
- Turkey breasts (avoid deli meats; they are high in sodium and low in protein)
- Water-packed Tuna
- White fish
- Eggs
- Halibut
- Cod
- Round steak
- Top sirloin

FATS

- Flaxseed Oil

SUPPLEMENTS

- Vitamin and mineral formula
- Vitamin C
- Chromium picolinate
- Fish oil capsules (if you don't use flaxseed oil)
- Meal replacement powders (such as Prolab's Lean Mass Matrix)
- Whey protein powders
- Protein bars
- Creatine
- Glutamine

DAIRY

- Skim Milk

MISCELLANEOUS ITEMS

- Garlic powder (for flavoring)
- Onion powder (for flavoring)
- Balsamic vinegar
- Crystal light
- Any sugar-free and salt-free seasoning

(Photocopy these pages for your own personal use)

Body Hair Free

H

THE **BODY SCULPTING BIBLE** FOR **MEN**

ELIMINATING BODY HAIR

This particular section is dedicated to a topic that many men either don't think about or, because of the "masculinity" thing, believe they shouldn't think about. The topic we're talking about is body hair and whether or not you should shave it or, at least, trim it. Now, I understand that there are men and women out there who like and even love body hair. For all of you that do in fact enjoy the hairy side of life, this is not a plea to change your personal preference. It is merely a "How To" guide created to help those who would like to make a change.

When I was a young man, I never thought about shaving my body hair. The reasons for this were simple. First, I really didn't have much hair to begin with and second, I was fat! Speaking for myself and for many heavy people, the last thing a heavy person wants to do is reveal their naked body. Whether it is with the help of the clothes we wear or the body hair we accumulate over time, we would much rather try and hide from what we aren't comfortable with showing.

Over the years I began working out and, as a result, began depleting my body fat while simultaneously building lean muscle mass. I knew I was losing fat because my fat calipers indicated so. I knew I was gaining muscle because the tape measure showed an increase in my measurements. That made me feel great but whenever I took off my shirt, I didn't look as good as I thought I would. This pushed me towards working even harder than ever but to no avail, I still wasn't pleased. I got to the point where I became obsessed with working out and ended up pushing too hard. In fact, I pushed so hard that I began physically injuring myself. Furthermore, it didn't even help with my appearance.

One day, at the age of 18, I bought a copy of a fitness magazine called MuscleMag. I discovered that these guys looked amazing and not one of

them had body hair! That's how I wanted to look. Without the body hair, you could clearly see all of the hard work these guys put in to working out. I began to think. What if I shaved? Will it look right on me? I concluded that it just wouldn't look right on me. With that thought, I didn't shave for the next three years.

When I finally did decide to shave, I did so with a disposable razor and shaving cream. I was merely experimenting so I started with my chest only. At first, I really didn't like it. I looked and felt like a little kid. About two weeks later, I decided to shave my stomach.

Believe me when I tell you that it looks much better when both are shaved, rather than having a bare chest and a hairy stomach.

All of a sudden I could see my abs and, although I knew I had great abs there somewhere, I could finally see a six-pack! It was like they had just suddenly appeared. I looked at my chest again and noticed that I had these muscle striations and deep cuts in my chest region. All I could think was: "Where the heck did these come from?" At that point, the shocking realization was that, for the three years prior to me shaving, this same body existed. Wow, I actually had really looked like this for about three years! Can you believe that? For three years I could have taken off my shirt at the beach and had people admiring my body. I could have felt confident and who knows how much further I could have come during that time.

I've told this story to many people since my discovery and many of them felt that this story was perhaps exaggerated. The suggestion that I suddenly noticed that I had this nice body seemed far-fetched. I posed this question to them and to you now: Why do you think all of those fitness or supplement companies are so successful when running those "before and after" pictorial fitness contests? I'm sure you've seen them before. They are before and after picture campaigns where the featured men are all plump, pasty and hairy in their before pictures. In these men's after pictures though, did you happen to notice that they are all tanned up in addition to being hairless? Of course, you must give credit where credit is due and admit that some of these men have made some very admirable changes to their physiques. While this is true for some, the majority of these pictures depict improvements made possible with the help of suntan lotions and a razor.

Why do you think these companies would have their male contestants shave and go tanning before they took their after pictures? Let's be honest, many of you have been complimented when you've gotten a tan. When we're tan, we often get compliments regarding our "nice color" or our seemingly "thinner frame". A tan obviously makes us LOOK much better than when we're pale. A tan can help us look more vibrant, more toned and yes, even more muscular. The companies that hold these fitness contests are smart to make these powerful improvements to their contestants' physiques.

The point here is that you can also help improve your physical appearance when you are tan. If you are concerned about your health regarding overexposure to the sun, there are many new and safe tanning methods including, but not limited to, self-tanning lotions.

Do some research and explore the many options available to you.

As far as eliminating body hair is concerned, there are many options from which you can choose. The first method we will speak of is the traditional method of shaving with a razor. Trying out this particular method should be based on how sensitive your skin is to shaving. If you have a history of skin problems or a tendency to getting skin irritations when you shave your face, you should probably avoid this option. I personally have sensitive skin and do not prefer this method of body hair elimination. Shaving

with a razor can also greatly increase your chances of getting ingrown hairs. In addition to these potential problems, shaving with a razor can be time consuming. If you do decide to go with this method, go slow and apply some type of skin conditioning cream on your shaved body parts when you've finished.

The second method of shaving, and my personal favorite, is trimming the body hair with a hair buzzer. I recommend a hair buzzer that has a built in hair length mechanism, which will allow you to quickly and easily increase or decrease the amount of hair you would like to buzz away. Keep in mind that the best results will appear when you buzz in the opposite direction that the hair is growing in. Even if your goal is not to get a close buzz, shaving in the opposite direction of hair growth will allow you to achieve an even buzz cut. As you're buzzing away the hair, you might notice that the hair accumulates in the hair length mechanism and razor heads. Be aware that this can inhibit the buzzer from cutting evenly and can cause the buzzer head to yank hair from the root. This can be painful so make sure to hold the buzzer upside down and clean out the hair every so often. You can complete your entire body very quickly using this method of hair elimination and usually without any chance of skin irritation. Just remember that there is no need to push the buzzer abrasively along the skin. You might have to go over some areas more than once or twice but remember to use light, even strokes.

The third method of body hair elimination, and one you must be careful in trying out, is the hair removal lotions. I can't stress to you enough how careful you must be when using this method, as misuse or even slight carelessness can cause bad irritations and even burns. You must pay attention to the amount of time you're suppose to leave the lotion on. If you leave it on for a longer period of time than recommended, you risk being burned. Usually, these lotions call for dabbing large amounts of the lotion over the body while avoiding sensitive areas. Usually, they indicate to only leave the lotion on for fifteen minutes. You then get a damp washcloth and wipe the hair right off your body. You might be recommended to apply a skin conditioning lotion when complete. To make you understand how careful you must be with these lotions, I will tell you about my experience with a hair removal lotion. I did exactly what the lotions instructions indicated. I tested the lotion on my chest and tried to make sure that I avoided my nipples. When the recommended fifteen minutes were up, I immediately grabbed a damp washcloth and wiped the hair from my chest. It was working but I did start to experience some burning sensations in my chest area. Remember, fifteen minutes was the maximum time I was allowed to leave the lotion on for. I was in a race to wipe off the lotion and must have accidentally gotten some on my nipples. Now, in that moment I truly did not realize just how serious it could be getting even a trace of that lotion on my nipple area. The next day I had a blister on my nipple and some bad irritation on the skin of my chest. Still, I went to the gym and, when I started to sweat, OH MY GOSH! My chest and nipples burned so bad that I can't even describe it. Two days later, I had a fairly large scab on my left nipple. As you can see, even after carefully following the directions, you can still run into problems with these products. You must be very careful not to take the cautions lightly. Please pay close attention to the directions and monitor your application of the lotions at all times.

The fourth method, and one that I refuse to ever try again, is waxing. It is by far the most painful method I know for eliminating body hair. I've heard all the different claims stating how this and that waxing system is a pain free means to removing unwanted body hair. Well, apparently the people making those claims have not tried waxing themselves or perhaps their pain receptors in their body were numb when they did try it. Regardless, waxing, my friends, is painful. But hey, if you can handle the pain, go for it! If you can withstand the pain of waxing, it will provide you with one of the smoothest results you will get from all of the body hair removal methods we've mentioned so far.

The last two methods we will mention are for you to research yourself. They are the Electrolysis method and Laser hair removal methods. Both can be expensive and require a medical doctor or licensed technician to perform. Either ask your dermatologist to refer you to a practitioner or look in the phone book for a list of local offices.

As you can see, you have many options to choose from when it comes to body hair elimination. If I were to make a suggestion, I would suggest that you first try the buzzer method since it is the most mild of the methods.

I should point something out to you before you get too excited about removing your body hair. If this is the first time you've ever started working out and wish to shave because you think you'll look much better than you do now, please don't mislead yourself. If it's simply a matter of removing the hair because you really don't like it, then by all means do so. However, don't do it expecting to look like someone who has been working out for a long time. Too many people have strong expectations of what they should look like and can easily get discouraged when they don't see what they thought they would see. You need to be thick-skinned and face the fact that you need to work out, eat well and pay your dues in order to look the way you want. When you do begin to work hard and pay attention to all of the variables that help to create a healthy and fit lifestyle, it would not be surprising to see that your results end up being much better than

even those high expectations of what you originally thought you'd look like.

If I were you and were just starting out with
the fitness lifestyle, I would not shave my body
hair right now. I would set a goal for myself
and look forward to seeing those goals met.
When you're ready, you'll know the right time
to eliminate that body hair and when you do,
WOW! You'll be amazed at yourself. Think of it
as an unveiling ceremony.

Yeah it might seem a little corny, but you'll
be the only one laughing.

Appendix I
Body Sculpting Under Special Circumstances

I

THE **BODY**
SCULPTING
BIBLE
FOR **MEN**

BODY SCULPTING FOR OLDER MEN

During the past several years, many point to the many benefits and safety of weight training exercise for aging adults. Among these benefits are the usual benefits of reduced cholesterol, reduced blood pressure, reduced resting pulse rate, increased levels of muscle mass, increased levels of bone density and decreased levels of body fat. In addition to those benefits, weight training for older men offers the following:

• Improved digestion.

• Improved blood glucose levels.

• Reduced discomfort caused by arthritis.

• Reduced lower back pain.

• Increased mobility (due to an increase in muscle strength).

• Reduced possibility of a fall due to loss of balance caused by loose joints and weak leg muscles.

In order for older men to get all of the benefits that strength training has to offer the following guidelines must be followed:

First and foremost, consult with your doctor and/or physical therapist before you start any exercise program. Depending on your present condition, you may or may not need someone to supervise you during your weight training session. If you have been physically active all your life, you should have no problems going full bore into a weight training routine. If, you have never been very physically active and you suffer from ailments like loss of balance, then supervision will be required.

Educate yourself on how to perform the exercises correctly! Read the exercise description section in this book as many times as necessary. Study the illustrations and practice the movement mentally. It is crucial that exercise form is followed in order to avoid injury.

Ensure that you follow the nutritional guidelines of our Nutrition Chapter. Many senior citizens in this country are malnourished, as their appetites have decreased over the years. Also, certain medications cause a loss of appetite as well. Force yourself to follow our nutrition guidelines and we guarantee that you won't be malnourished. Remember that in order to get the maximum effect from training, the diet has to be in order. Being malnourished leads to a loss of muscle mass (the body is using such mass as fuel) and a resulting loss of strength and bone density (which leads to brittle bones).

You have two choices for the exercise program. If you have always been physically active and you are in good health, go ahead and start with our Break-In Routine and progress to the 14-Day Body Sculpting Workout. If on the other hand, you suffer from ailments like loss of balance and have perhaps limited mobility, use the following program that is composed of machines:

DAY 1

• Leg Extensions

• Seated Leg Curls

• Leg Press

• Calf Press

• Lower Back Machine

• Abdominal Machine

DAY 2

- Pulldown to Front
- Close-Grip Pulldown
- Overhead Press Machine
- Rear-Delt Machine
- Biceps Curl Machine
- Triceps Extension Machine

HOW TO PROGRESS

- Follow the same structure of the 14-Day Body Sculpting Workout;

- Use weights on Mon/Wed/Fri alternating between Day 1 and 2.

- Do cardio on Tue/Thu/ Saturday.

- Sundays are for complete rest.

- Weeks 1-2: Perform 2 sets of 15 to 18 repetitions per exercise. Take 2 seconds to lift the weight and 4 to lower it. Rest 1 minute in between sets. No weight training techniques such as modified compound supersets are to be utilized. Perform one set after the other in straight set fashion.

- Weeks 3-4: Increase to 3 sets of 12 to 15 repetitions. Take 2 seconds to lift the weight and 4 to lower it. Rest 1 minute in between sets. No weight training techniques such as modified compound supersets are to be utilized. Perform one set after the other in straight set fashion.

- Weeks 5-6: Go up to 4 sets of 10-12 repetitions. Take 2 seconds to lift the weight and 4 to lower it. Rest 1 minute in between sets. No weight training techniques such as modified compound supersets are to be uti-

lized. Perform one set after the other in straight set fashion.

- On cardio days, build up to 25 minutes of continuous aerobic exercise performed at 70-75 percent of your maximum heart rate. Start with 5 minutes of aerobics 3 times a week, and add 2 minutes every week to the original 5 minutes. At the end of 10 weeks you should be able to do 25 minutes of continuous aerobic exercise with no problems. Use Sundays as your complete rest day from diet and exercise. If after a while of using this routine you feel that you are in shape to do the 14-Day Body Sculpting Routine, then by all means do so by using the exercises listed above. If you feel that you are ready to incorporate some free weight exercises as well, then go for it!

YOUNGSTERS AND WEIGHT TRAINING

At what age a teenage boy can start working out with weights has always been a topic of debate. Some people say that weights should not be touched until after all of the growing is done or else you could affect the growth platelets and stunt your growth. Others say it is okay to start lifting weight at an early age. We have arrived at the following conclusions based on the latest research on this subject.

We believe that youngsters (anybody **less than 12 years old**) are better off doing exercises with just their body weight. The following exercises should compose a youngster's program:

- Running
- Dips
- Push-ups
- Pull-ups

- Chin-ups
- Squats with no weights
- Lunges with no weights
- Calf raises with no weight
- Crunches
- Leg raises

Depending on the age and motivation of the person, anywhere between 2-5 sets of each exercise for the maximum amount of reps possible is sufficient. There should be 30 seconds of rest in between exercises and they should be performed 3 times a week.

An additional 15-20 minutes of running on their rest day is enough exercise for anyone who wishes to start an exercise program before the age of 13.

13-year-olds can start working out with weights as long as they're using weights light enough to allow 20-30 reps per set. They should basically follow the same program described above with the same set, repetition and rest scheme, plus adding the following dumbbell exercises: dumbbell curls, dumbbell overhead triceps extensions, and lateral raises. In addition, dumbbells can also be used to perform lunges, squats and calf raises. The complete program will look like the following:

- Running
- Dips
- Push-ups
- Pull-ups
- Chin-ups
- Lateral raises
- Dumbbell curls
- Dumbbell overhead triceps extensions

- Dumbbell squats
- Dumbbell lunges
- Dumbbell calf raises
- Crunches
- Leg raises

Continue this program for the next three years.

15-year-olds can start increasing the weight but should stay within 13-20 reps. For the next two years they should concentrate on perfecting their exercise technique and form. They must make sure to only increase the weight when they can do over 20 repetitions easily. They should not go to absolute muscular failure or use any fancy weight training techniques, since there is still some bone growth and development occurring in their bodies. Remember, strenuous and heavy weighted exercise can interfere with the growth process, so keep it simple!

At this age it is okay to use the 14-Day Body Sculpting routines from this book as long as the 13-20 repetition rule is kept (Weeks 1-2: 18-20 reps are used, weeks 3-4: 16-18, weeks 5-6: 13-15).

After 18, you can start going heavier in weight with no problems; by then all of the growth platelets, bone and joint structure should be fully developed.

FITNESS WHILE TRAVELING

We always use traveling as an excuse to not get in shape. Getting in shape while traveling is more challenging, but it is certainly possible. Provided that you are determined, the key is planning and preparation. We have taught all of our clients to learn to treat exercise as a way of life. This way, you are innately drawn to exercising even during vacation time. We have gotten some of the best workouts of our lives during vacation and traveling. It is refreshing to go to train in new environments and surroundings, plus a great way to meet people.

Before you go on your next trip, find out if the hotel that you are going to stay in has a fitness facility or at least a set of dumbbells. If not, then find out where the closest fitness facility is and plan to work out there. If, by some twist of fate, there are no fitness facilities in the area (hard to believe), then try to do the youngsters weight training routine which consists of dips, push-ups, pull-ups, chin-ups, squats with no weights, lunges with no weights, calf raises with no weight, crunches and leg raises performed 3 times a week for 5 sets with 30 seconds of rest in between sets of as many reps as possible. Run for 20-30 minutes first thing in the morning on rest days. All you need for this routine is a park with a chin-up bar and parallel bars. If there is no park within the area, then you can still do push-ups, pull-ups, chin-ups, squats with no weights, lunges with no weights, calf raises with no weight, crunches and leg raises. All you need to carry is a portable chin-up bar that you can place in the hotel room. Once you get back home, you can start doing the 14-Day Body Sculpting Workout as laid out with the only exception being that you should start it on Week 3, since you have already done high repetition, light weight work.

With diet, you will need to get creative. Follow the rules from the section on eating out. Also, carry with you protein bars so that you are prepared with all of the required meals for the day. Missing meals too often guarantees failure with this program.

As you can see, even though it will take more effort to get in shape if you travel, it is not impossible. If you are determined enough to change your body, then nothing is impossible!

TRAINING WHILE YOU ARE SICK

Nothing can bring progress to a halt more than when you are sick. We are often asked the question, should I train while I am sick? The answer to that question really depends on what you mean by sick. Is it a cold? The flu? Allergies? Most people confuse the common cold for the flu. However, these are different types of illnesses. The flu is caused by viruses known as Influenza A or Influenza B, while the common cold is caused by viruses called coronaviruses and rhinoviruses. There are over 200 different types of coronaviruses and rhinoviruses. If one of them hits you, your immune system builds a lifelong immunity to it (therefore, the same virus will never hit you twice). However, you have the rest of the viruses that have not yet affected you to worry about; and there are enough to last a lifetime.

The flu, as you may have already found out by experience, is much more severe as it is usually accompanied by an array of body aches and fever. Therefore, your body's immune system is taxed much more by the flu than by the common cold. At this time, training would not only be detrimental to muscle growth, but it would also be very detrimental to your health as well. Remember that while training can help us gain muscle, lose fat, feel good and energetic, it is still a catabolic activity. The body needs to be in good health in order to go from the catabolic state caused by the exercise to an anabolic state of recuperation and muscle growth. So if you have the flu, your body is already fighting a catabolic state caused by the Influenza virus. In this case, weight training would only add more catabolism, which in turn would negatively affect the efficacy of the immune system against the virus, causing you to get sicker. Therefore, absolutely no training if you have the flu. Instead, concentrate on very good nutrition and on drinking large amounts of fluids (water and electrolyte replacement drinks like Gatorade in order to prevent dehydration). Once the flu completely runs its course, you can slowly start up the 14-Day Body Sculpting Workout on week 1 starting with light weights. Don't push yourself too hard during this first week. The next week you'll repeat week 1 again, but pushing yourself closer to muscular failure. By the second week of the program you should be back on track.

If it is the common cold that is hitting you and the particular virus is mild (you know that it is mild when your symptoms are just a runny nose and slight coughing), you may get away with training as long as you stop the sets short of reaching muscular failure and you decrease the weight poundages by 25 percent (divide the weights that you usually use by 4 and that will give you the amount of weight that you need to take off the bar) in order to prevent you from pushing too hard. Again, if the cold virus is causing you to feel run down, achy, with a sore throat and headaches, it would be best to stop training all together, until the symptoms subside. If this is the case, just follow the exercise program start-up recommendations described above for after the flu. Remember that we do not want to make it any harder for the immune system to fight the virus by introducing more catabolic activity, so intense training is out during that time.

If your ailment is something other than the common cold or the flu, consult your doctor.

Now that we have seen how a flu or a cold can throw a wrench into your progress, let's see how we can prevent these buggers from affecting us during the flu season or during any other season for that matter.

While it is still unknown why the cold and flu season generally comes during the winter months, it is known that you have to let the virus into your system in order for it to affect you. Therefore, it is only logical that we implement a two-fold prevention approach:

Prevent the virus from infiltrating your system. Keeping in mind that cold viruses spread by human contact, that they get into your system through the mouth, eyes and nose, and that they can remain active for up to three hours, you can accomplish this by doing the following:

- Keep your hands away from your face

- Wash your hands with anti bacterial soap frequently throughout the day (especially as soon as you finish your workout at the gym).

Maintain immune system operation at peak efficiency levels at all times. Remembering that excessive exercise, a bad diet, and losing sleep are all catabolic activities, do the following:

- Avoid overtraining by using the principles advocated in this book.

- Maintain a balanced diet as described in the nutrition chapter and avoid processed foods that contain high levels of saturated fats, refined flours or sugar since these types of foods lower the immune system function.

- Get a healthy dose of sleep a day (anywhere from 7 to 9 hours depending on your individual requirements).

So remember, stay healthy by following the tips above, and if you get sick, then "don't beat a tired horse" as former Mr. Olympia Lee Haney used to say. Rest until you get better! If you don't you will end up more seriously ill and this will take you out of the gym for a longer period of time.

Appendix J
Anatomy Charts

THE **BODY**
SCULPTING
BIBLE
FOR **MEN**

J

MALE MUSCULAR AND SKELETAL ANATOMY

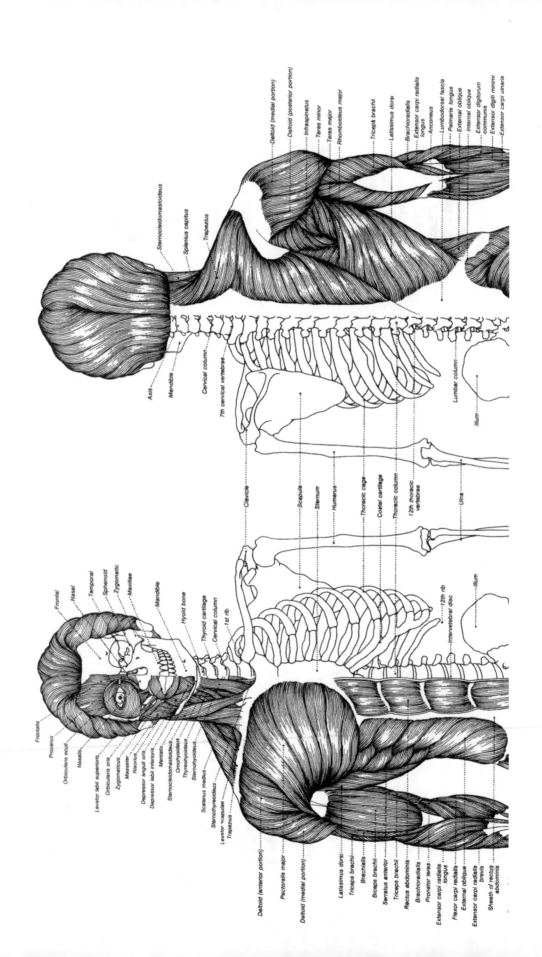

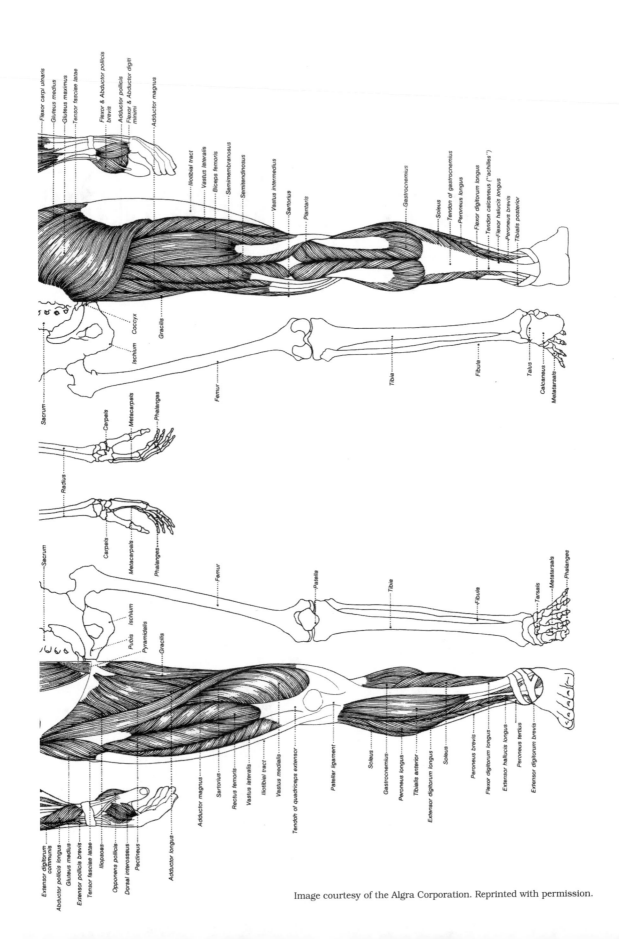

Image courtesy of the Algra Corporation. Reprinted with permission.

Exercise Descriptions

THE BODY SCULPTING BIBLE FOR MEN

PROPER EXERCISE TECHNIQUE

Learning proper exercise technique is the backbone of every fitness program. If you train improperly you will not stimulate the intended muscle, and will risk major injury as well as receiving little or no results. When you learn to use proper exercise technique you will receive twice the results in half the time, guaranteed! We see people in the gym day in and day out who have no idea how to properly train their muscles. Some of them are professional bodybuilders, some are professional athletes, and some are even certified fitness trainers. Unfortunately, the ones who really suffer the most are people like you who rely on these role models for wisdom and guidance. We will show you the proper exercise technique to use for optimal results. Just remember to utilize your newfound knowledge. Like the old saying, "Feed a man a fish and he'll eat for a day, teach a man to fish and he'll eat for a lifetime." We expect the same of you. We don't want you to read this book once and forget everything you've learned. We want you to learn and utilize that knowledge to achieve astounding results.

Applying proper exercise form and technique is without doubt the most important component of any fitness program. Without it, many setbacks will occur. First, the musculature you intend to exercise will not be stimulated as efficiently as possible. Exercise should not be focused around just lifting barbells and weights. It shouldn't just be about how much you can lift. Optimum fitness is about the quality of exercise, the quality of your form and how you maintain that form, especially during heavier lifting. Proper exercise technique coupled with the Zone-Tone principle that we presented in **Chapter 1** will bring you the most astonishing results with the minimum amount of sets. Why? Because as we

have already discussed, one properly executed set is equivalent to five sets of "just going through the motions" type of exercise. *It comes down to this; if you want to get the most out of your workout, keep the intensity high without sacrificing proper form.* Neglecting to focus on proper form quickly leads to no results, while practicing perfect proper form equals incredible results quickly!

WHICH EXERCISES ARE THE BEST FOR FAST RESULTS?

In weight training, there are a variety of exercises that one can choose from to sculpt the body of your dreams. Results in bodybuilding or body sculpting are generally measured in body composition changes; increased muscle mass or tone, depending on the goal, along with decreases in body fat. The speed at which such changes are acquired depends on the training protocol used, the nutrition plan followed and the amount of rest that the trainee gets. In order for a training protocol to work at peak efficiency, not only must it be periodized or cycled but it also must include exercises that give you the most stimulation in the minimum amount of time.

Different exercises provide different levels of stimulation. Exercises like leg extensions, while excellent for sculpting the lower part of the quadriceps, produce less of a stimulating effect than an exercise like the squat. The efficacy of an exercise really depends on the exercise's ability to involve the maximum amount of muscle fibers and also on its ability to provide a neuromuscular stimulation (NMS). Neuromuscular stimulation is of crucial importance as it is the nervous system that ultimately sends a signal to the brain requesting to start the muscle growth process. How do we determine what the stimulation factor of each exercise is?

THE NMS CLASSES

In order to rate what the NMS of each exercise is, we borrowed the Class rating system used for classifying the speed of DSL systems (the technology used to achieve high speed connections to the Internet through your phone line) and tailored it to fit our purpose. In this system a Class 1 technology has lower speeds than a Class 2 technology. Therefore, in our exercise rating system composed of four classes, a Class 1 exercise yields the lowest NMS (this class is composed of variable resistance machine type exercises) while a Class 4 exercise yields the highest NMS and is therefore the hardest but most stimulating one. In each class we may also have subclasses such as Class 1a and Class 1b. A Class 1a exercise will yield less NMS than a Class 1b.

Class 1a exercises are composed of isolation (one joint) exercises performed in variable resistance machines (such as Nautilus) where the whole movement of the exercise is controlled. These type of exercises provide the least amount of stimulation as stabilizer muscles do not need to get involved since the machine takes care of the stabilization process. An example of such an exercise would be the machine curl.

Class 1b exercises are compound (multi-joint) movements performed in a variable resistance machine. An example of such movement would be the incline bench press performed in a Hammer Strength machine. Since the movement is a compound one, more muscles get involved and therefore the neuromuscular stimulation is higher than that offered by a machine curl. However, the fact that the machine takes care of the stabilization issues limits the growth offered by the exercise.

Class 2a exercises are composed of isolation (one joint) exercises performed with non-variable resistance machines. An example of such exercise would be the leg extension exercise performed in one of those leg extensions attachments that come with the benches that are sold for home gyms. These attachments lack the pulleys and the cams that would make the exercise a variable resistance exercise. Therefore, the muscles need to get more involved in the movement, providing better stimulation.

Class 2b exercises are composed of basic (multi-joint) exercises performed with non-variable resistance machines. An example of such would be the bench press unit that is attached to the Universal type of machines or a leg press machine that contains no pulleys or cams that would make the exercise easier. Since there are no pulleys or cams to make the exercise easier as you lift the weight, the NMS is higher.

Class 3a exercises are isolation (one joint) exercises performed with free weights. An example of such exercise would be a concentration curl performed with a dumbbell. It is still not very clear whether a multi joint exercise performed on a machine offers the same amount or better NMS than the one offered by a free weight isolation exercise. However, for the purposes of this discussion, we will assume that the free weight isolation exercise provides more stimulation as stabilizer muscles come into play (especially if you do the exercise standing up).

Class 3b exercises are multi-jointed basic exercises performed with barbell free weights.

Class 3c exercises are multi-jointed basic exercises performed with dumbbell free weights. The barbell exercises provide less NMS as the movement is more restrained as opposed to dumbbells where the weights can go in all directions unless all of your stabilizer muscles jump in and constrain the movement. Because of this, dumbbells provide the highest NMS in this category.

Finally, Class 4 exercises are free weight exercises where your body moves through space. In other words, any exercise where your torso is the one moving, such as squats, deadlifts, pull-ups, close grip chins, pushups, lunges, and dips, will provide the most stimulation possible and therefore, the fastest results. Haven't you seen at the gym how many people do great amounts of weights in a pulldown machine but have trouble doing pull-ups? The reason for this is that in order for you to perform these type of exercises you need to be capable of not only carrying the added resistance but also involving your body-weight as well. Therefore, many muscles are called into play in order to perform this feat. Performing dips, chinups, squats and deadlifts you are really hitting every single muscle in your body! These exercises not only give you fast results, but they also create functional strength; in other words strength that can be used for your daily activities. If you are great at performing pull-ups and you go to perform a pulldown you'll see how easy the task of performing a pulldown is. As a matter of fact, depending on your pull-up strength, you might be able to lift the whole stack in most pulldown machines. However, the reverse is not

true. While you may be very good at performing pulldowns you may not be able to perform many pull-ups as the strength gained in the pulldown exercise is not as transferable as the one gained in a pull-up. Again, the reason for this phenomenon is NMS.

CONCLUSION

Now that you know what exercises are the ones that give you the most bang for your buck, my recommendations are as follows:

- If you follow the normal *14 Day Body Sculpting Workout* stick to Class 3 and 4 region exercises.

- If you follow the *Advanced 14 Day Body Sculpting Workout* you can get away with having 1/3 of your routine composed of lower class (Classes 2 and below) exercises.

Remember, convincing your body to grow and develop muscle is not an easy task. However it becomes an impossible one if you choose exercises that do not provide a significant NMS effect. Therefore, always choose exercises from the higher classes in order to show your body that you mean business.

FINAL THOUGHTS

The techniques presented in the sections above combined with the 14-Day Body Sculpting Training and Nutrition Principles, along with the knowledge presented on how to use your mind to improve your results at the gym and in anything else you do in life are what separate the 14-Day Body Sculpting Workout from anything you have ever read.

After reading this book you should have the knowledge necessary to control the way your body looks. Knowledge is power and the power to change the way your body looks will give you a sense of control that will spill over into other areas of your life. Soon you will discover that the discipline you use to re-sculpt your body can be used to accomplish any other goal that you want to reach in life. Now stop wishing and start doing! Go for it!

About the Authors

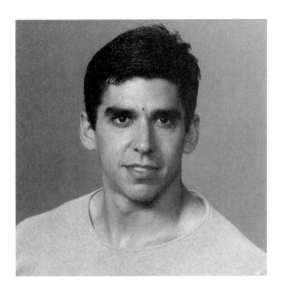

Hugo A. Rivera, ISSA Certified Personal Trainer and University of South Florida graduate with a Bachelor of Science in Engineering, was born in Bayamon, Puerto Rico. As an overweight child he experienced at an early age the feelings of insecurity that come with obesity. After becoming anorexic at the age of 13 and losing a total of 70 pounds in less than a year, his concerned parents took him to a nutritionist in an effort to stop the anorexic cycle. This nutritionist mentioned one thing that would change Hugo's outlook on dieting forever: "Eating food will not make you fat; only abusing the quantities of the bad foods

will." Hugo decided to kick his anorexia and to dedicate his life to studying the effects of foods on the human physiology.

By age 15, Hugo's interest in how food affects the shape and the form of your body naturally led to an interest in exercise and he became an avid natural bodybuilder.

Discovering early on that there wasn't much realistic or practical bodybuilding or fitness advice, he started to record what worked and what didn't for him. After much trial and error, he started finding principles that he noticed worked on any healthy human being. The best part of it all was his discovery that it is not necessary to spend all day at the gym in order to get results! Upset at the fact that many people in the industry did not care about trainees actually reaching their goals, he decided to create a web site and conducted personal training during his college years in an effort to spread all of the knowledge that he had acquired.

Ten years later Hugo is considered an expert in the industry and he has dedicated much of his time to helping normal people achieve their dream figures by sharing sensible and practical knowledge that he has found to work even

on the most stubborn metabolisms. His knowledge of human physiology and anatomy, combined with the analytical skills he developed in his engineering profession, enable him to produce extremely efficient programs that anyone can fit into their schedule. The fact that he was overweight and then extremely skinny (after the anorexic period) enables him to identify with all groups of people that have weight problems. He holds a steady engineering job as well as a successful personal training business, enabling him to offer practical advice to people with hectic lifestyles.

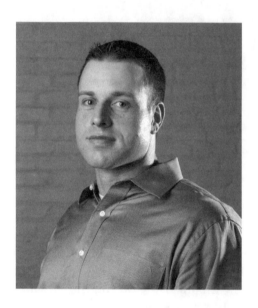

James Villepigue, ISSA Certified Personal Trainer, New York College of Oriental Medicine graduate of Massage Therapy and Hofstra University of New York graduate with a Bachelor of Science Degree in Marketing, was born May 20, 1971, in Roslyn, New York.

If you came across James at the ages of 10 through 17, the last thing you would think of was that he would be involved with health and fitness. Weighing 250 pounds at age 15, James

was anything but healthy and fit. Of course a genetic condition, like a thyroid deficiency, was not to blame. James simply had a love for indulging in his favorite foods, as most people do in America.

Like most people, he didn't know when to stop, and certainly never considered the consequences of eating so much. Throughout high school, James was bullied and ridiculed, to the point that he wanted to leave school permanently. Family members convinced him to stay and stick it out. But, every day he was forced to defend himself both mentally and physically. James was not a tough kid, did not like confrontation of any sort, and was at a point in his life where he desperately needed help. This was the turning point and the beginning of James Villepigue's involvement with weight training.

James has now been involved with the health and fitness industries for 10 years. He has certifications from the International Sports Sciences Association (ISSA) as a personal fitness trainer/counselor and from AFAA as a personal fitness trainer/counselor and weight room certified trainer. He was also appointed as a Strength and Conditioning Coach for the United States Karate Team. James also holds two United States Patents and one Canadian Patent for a revolutionary piece of exercise/medical equipment called "Digiciser".

Throughout his career, James has passionately kept up to date with the latest trends and rapid changes within the bodybuilding and fitness world. The adversity that once accompanied his life is not unlike the lives of so many teenagers and adults today. This, combined with his appreciation for his ability to create success out of his struggles, led him to dedicate his life to helping others make their fitness dreams and goals come true. When James thinks about his life now, he is grateful for the direction in which it has taken him, as he can now identify with anyone who struggles with eating disorders and adversity. Today, James Villepigue is a world-class fitness and bodybuilding trainer whose accomplishments have made him top in his class.

GOT QUESTIONS? NEED ANSWERS? THEN GO TO:

www.bodysculptingbible.com

IT'S FITNESS 24/7

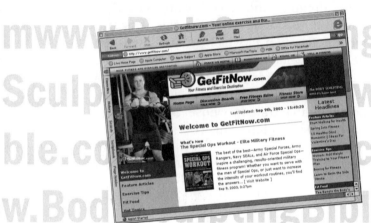

NEWS & TIPS

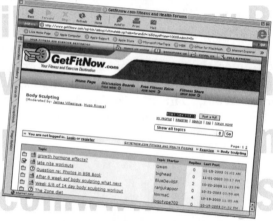

DISCUSSION GROUPS

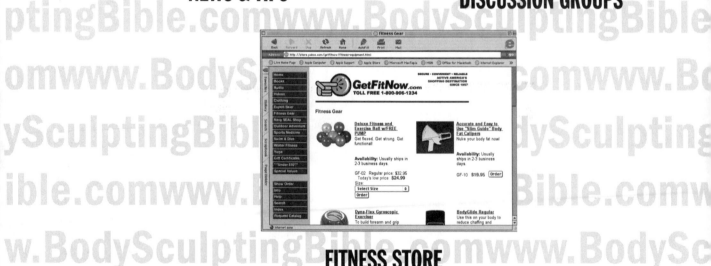

FITNESS STORE

It's a powerful resource for anyone seeking advice knowledge and more.
Visit today and sign up for our **FREE** newsletter.

Powered by **GETFITNOW.com**

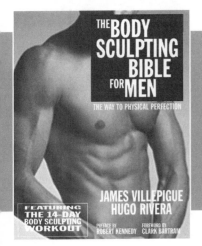
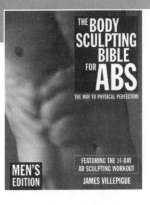
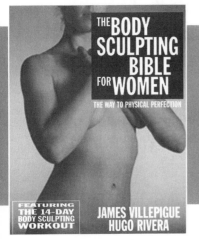
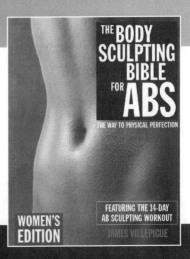

Also available

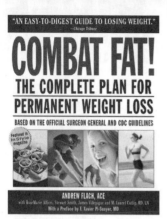

COMBAT FAT!

Combat Fat! puts you in charge of your weight loss goals with its motivating, step-by-step 8-week plan

$15.95

ISBN 1-58726-119-8

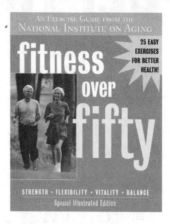

FITNESS OVER FIFTY

The National Institute on Aging's ultimate guide to staying fit and healthy for those over 50.

$15.95

ISBN 1-57826-136-8

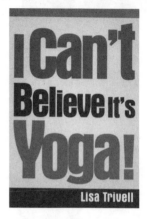

I CAN'T BELIEVE IT'S YOGA!

Lisa Trivell, one of the top yoga instructors in the U.S., finds fun new ways to bring yoga into our lives... American-style!

$14.95

ISBN 1-58726-032-9

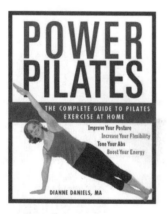

POWER PILATES

An Excellent way to build core strength and increase your aerobic endurance.

$15.95

ISBN 1-57826-147-3

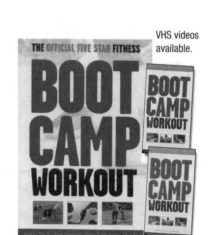

VHS videos available.

The Official Five Star Fitness BOOT CAMP WORKOUT

The most complete, instructive, and challenging workout ever devised. No major equipment nor health club membership required.

$14.95

ISBN 1-57826-033-7